It's Time To Sing My Song

Overcoming Circumstances with Faith

by
M. Marva Allison

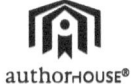

authorHOUSE®

AuthorHouse™
1663 Liberty Drive, Suite 200
Bloomington, IN 47403
www.authorhouse.com
Phone: 1-800-839-8640

First published by AuthorHouse 11/21/2007

ISBN: 978-1-4343-0081-2 (sc)

Printed in the United States of America
Bloomington, Indiana

This book is printed on acid-free paper.

Unless otherwise indicated, all scripture quotations are taken from
King James Version of the Bible.

Direct quotations from the Bible appear in bold type.

Then your light shall break forth

like the dawn, and your healing

shall spring up quickly;

your vindicator shall go

before you, the glory of the

LORD shall be your rear guard.

Then you shall call, and the LORD

will answer; you shall cry for help,and he will say,

Here I am.

- ISAIAH 58: 8,9

Dedi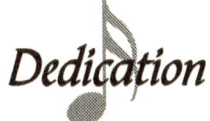cation

This book is dedicated to the loving memory of:

My beautiful parents, Preston and Mable Broussard, Sr. and the memory of my beloved brother, Walmon J. Broussard;

To my precious granddaughter, Lisette V. Allison; to my extended family; my prayer partners; and countless cancer survivors who have inspired me.

This book is dedicated to you.

To all the individuals who believe that God works in our lives and does answer prayers, this book is dedicated to you.

Acknowledgments

Some acknowledgments are in order:

To my heavenly Father, who holds me near and dear, thank you for never giving up on me despite my human weaknesses. You are everything that I need.

To my son, Regis Allison Jr., and his wife, Samantha, you have my undying gratitude for your relentless support, love, and effortless care. I love you, individually and collectively.

To my sister, Deborah, and my brother, Preston, thanks for the love, encouragement, and all the special memories that we as siblings share.

To your families, thanks for caring and sharing during these times. I love you all.

To my longtime girlfriend, confidante, and sister in Christ, Mary, when all else fails, I can turn to you. Thanks for your supporting counsel. We have a long history together. May we share many, many more.

To my special, traveling angel, and cousin, Betty Joe, words cannot express how grateful am I to you. Thanks for always being there. I love our "reach-out-and-touch" relationships.

To my Louisiana family, Edna, Lillian, Herman, Evelyn, Melba, Gen, Judie, Allen, Margo, all members of the Colston and White families, thanks for your words of encouragement, cards, prayers, and love.

To my Illinois family, Mrs. Mathis, Dorothy, Iva, Clyde, the Cades, the Burris, the Pitre, St. Ailbe's prayer partners, the Schaffers, Glenn, Buford, Janice, Patrice, Ms. Mitchell, Angela and all those who have prayed for my well being, thank you.

To Harold, thanks for helping me to believe in myself and sharing God's praises with me.

To my South Holland family, thanks for your time, prayers, and hope for the future.

To Mrs. Gray and my Georgia family, Sunday school class, and prayer partners, your telephone calls, cards, and friendship helped to anchor me in the storm.

To my writing angels, thank you for the insight into the "Word" that has affected my life and circumstance. Thanks for your time and effort you put into critiquing my project. Your belief in me helped me to keep writing. The effort you put into critiquing my project never fails to shine.

To Barbara and all my New York families and friends, thanks for all the wonderful things you taught me to expect and love.

To my doctors, nurses, technicians, caregivers, and the staff of Northwestern Medical Foundation, I am forever grateful for your vision, direction, care and medical services.

To the thousands of people who prayed for my recovery, I love and appreciate you.

To the American Cancer Association, thanks for your dedication, and all that you do to help all cancer patients, their families, and survivors.

To the staff of the Jennifer S. Fallick Cancer Support Center, thanks for all the programs, support groups and information that inspires all to "live better with cancer through community, sharing, and nurturing the mind, body, and spirit."

For all who took me under their wings, offered their unique points of view, shared their time and energy to go through this journey with me, may God continue to bless and keep you.

If any names were omitted, of anyone who has prayed for my sanity and recovery, please blame it on "senior moments," not my heart. May God continue to do great things for all.

Foreword

The year was 2002. The month was November. Learning that I had been diagnosed with breast cancer was quite a shock to my system and well-being. St. Paul said that, "All things work together for our good." In all things, situations, issues, problems, God is working for our good. Regardless of the good, bad, or ups and downs, he is involved. St. Paul did not say that God would not allow some circumstances and or situations to challenge my beliefs. He had not left me to chance or fate. God was working through me. He was actively involved in my life. As Pastor Jamal Bryant declared, "Something was about to happen in my atmosphere." This was not what I expected. It was not what I desired. Hey, I am just building my case.

Trust me. Upon receiving my diagnosis, this was not my emotional outlook. Fear, anxiety, anger, and depression were just some of the stages that I experienced. Not understanding what seemed like a death sentence at the time, I was frustrated and disappointed that my life seemed to be ending before I had accomplished some of my dreams. Knowing that God's promised life expectancy is based on the "three-scores" theory, I felt that I was being cheated. The emotional feelings, fear, anger, frustration, and uncertainty—which are considered "normal" by cancer experts—did not feel normal to me.

Let's go further. Hearing the words *you have cancer* (or the big "C") seemed like "nailing a death coffin shut." My battle was set. There were issues that had to be faced. At every stage, from diagnosis, surgery, reconstruction, treatments, and learning to cope with decisions that had to be made, the reactions are troublesome to the receiver of the news. Believe me, I was no different from other cancer survivors who have had this experience.

As harsh as those words were, the reality of having to face my circumstances awakened me to the fact that I was not a quitter. I have a "Father" who did not want me to die an early death. Having been educated in the parochial system as well as having grown up in a praying family, I believed in taking my problems to God in prayer. Even if it was hard for me to comprehend or figure out this problem, I knew that God would work it for my good. Trying not to lose my mind, the affirmation, *"Every need will be met,"* became my "rod and staff." It was true at times. When I was so certain that I could not withstand the treatments, doctor's appointments, or pain associated with breast cancer, this affirmation kept me aware of that the "Infinite Supplier" of all my needs was very able.

Paul Dean Jackson, of Glenside, Pennsylvania, said, "With Spirit, anything is possible; anything begins anew." Having breast cancer has left me "naked before the Lord." In a way, it reminded me that I needed to strengthen my relationship with God. What was once important in my life became my primary focus. Using the Words of God to change my negative attitude to a more positive one opened channels and allowed his grace to flow more abundantly into my life. As said in Psalms 31:3:

> *"You are indeed my rock and my fortress; for your name's sake, lead me and guide me."*

The Rev. Dr. Claudette Anderson Copeland said, "The disease was a way of shaking loose everything that was not necessary and leaving us with the best of what it means to be alive." None of my days are taken for granted. Verbally and silently, I continue to thank God and praise him for my health, family, and friends. When depression or self-pity parties entered my physic I used the Word of God to shake me free. I feel an enormous amount of gratitude for continued progress and recovery. Having combined faith and trust in God, how can I lose? Dr. Martin Luther King, Jr. once described faith in a powerful way. He said, "Faith is taking the first step even when you don't see the whole staircase."

As a breast cancer survivor, learning to cope and live are very important.

Giving praise and thanks to God, I am so grateful to be alive and to be counted as a cancer survivor. As I think back, I understand how the love and faith of my family, friends and prayer partners helped me to heal. Prayers have been and continue to be an important part of my recovery and survival. I have made a commitment to take one step at a time in being a healthier and happier me.

"I will give thanks to the Lord with my whole heart; I will tell of all your wonderful deeds."

Psalm 9:1

Contents

Introduction

I would like to tell you a story.

Actually, I would like to share an awesome journey with you and the experiences that I had along the way. Let's see. Where do I start? First, how often did I daydream about retiring or living a better and different life? How many times did I come to the end of my proverbial rope and played with the idea of just leaving it all behind? I'm sure that in today's world, some people whose lives seemed to be passing them by, or who have been diagnosed with a terminal disease such as cancer, long for a breakthrough or the best resources to handle the situation—as I did. Sensing that something must be done, but not being sure *what* to do became a problem. Attention on how to deal with this situation by focusing on the *who or how* to deal with the issue took longer than I thought. But I did know that it would not take care of itself. Emotionally and mentally, I was drained.

Making plans on how to face this dilemma and following my gut instinct, the purpose of this test had not become clear to me. Going through a test with breast cancer was not an easy journey. I did not understand the purpose of the trial. In order to recognize that something powerful was going to come out of this experience, I had to experience some storms. What I had seemed to forget was that this was not my battle. For a couple of months, I had allowed Satan to torment me beyond belief. I had forgotten the power of prayer. As soon as I began to realize that God was in charge and that only he could calm my fears, there were indications that the situation would get worse. Raising my spiritual level through the power of prayer, I began to pray "the Blood of Jesus" and the Holy Ghost on the inside of me to calm my doubts.

Just like the disciples on the boat, I was not by myself. He was riding the storm with me. Boy, was I glad to remember this truth!

When the storms of life started raging, I asked God to stand by me, and my hope was built. Leaning on the Word of God, holding on with all of my strength, I had something down inside that eased my fears. I told myself this seemed to be a physical problem, but it was tearing me up mentally too and needed my undivided attention. After trying to have a meaningful conversation with God and connecting spiritually, it was time to turn this over to God in prayer. I have learned that God will supply my every need.

> *"Seek first the kingdom of God…all things shall be added unto you."*
>
> (See Matthew 6:33.)

Looking back, my decision to keep my secret was foolish, but at the time, this was better for me. The truth was that my moments of indecision stemmed from my fear of the unknown. My fears kept me from thinking rationally. They also caused me to forget that only God is in charge. Frustrated and confused, I prayed and I asked God to make direct my path. James 5:16 says "the effectual fervent prayer of a righteous man availeth much." My red-hot petitions to God were on a seven-day, twenty-four-hour rally.

Once I was able to come out of the fog, I was able to get busy and confront my challenges. Devastated that after a diagnostic mammogram, I was informed that I had breast cancer. What were my breast cancer risk? Well,

- I really had not thought about this because I had refused to have a mammogram. Why? Because I had heard that it was painful and just did not believe in the procedure. Nor had I considered the other types of women who might be at risk, including those who are starting menopause after fifty-five are currently taking hormone therapy for menopause.
- More than 75 percent of breast cancers occur in women over fifty.

2

Nevertheless, by concentrating and planning my course of attack, I was on the road to recovery. My friend, Mary, my cousin Betty, my children, Regis and Samantha, my sister, Deborah, my brother, Preston, their families, a host of extended families and friends decided that we would pray for direction and healing.

Involvement in prayer, meditation and other activities that helped me to face my circumstances and improved the quality of life was my major source of comfort. In all of what I considered my tight spots: mastectomy, reconstruction, chemotherapy, radiation, loss of hair, joint pains, nerve damage, and all other related symptoms, pleading God's "Precious Blood to flow through every cell of my body, *It's Time to Sing my Song;the title of this book.*

I acknowledge that God gave me a breakthrough during one of the most uncertain times of my life. He brought into my life a cousin I had not met before. This person was to enter my life and play a very crucial role. Also, he allowed one of my oldest and dearest friends to start and end this journey with me, without complaint. On top of all this, through God's grace, I witnessed the birth of my first grandchild, Lisette.

> *"Blessed be the Lord, my Rock, who trains my hands for battle, my fingers for war."*
> *(See Psalms 144:1)*

Today, when I have an area of concern (which I sometimes do), I contact my doctor, pray about it and move on. Research has indicated that breast cancer rates are down and survivors, with proper medical attention, are living longer and better lives.

I have learned that breast cancer requires maintenance. I have learned that with life changes, it is important that I recognize what is important to maintain a healthful live and to strive to remain healthy. Every day is not all roses, but learning how to trust in God and faith in his words, I am going to have a healthful and productive life. Praise the Lord!

Crying for a minute, I had something down on the inside that eased my storms. In trouble, I just said, "Jesus, my chief cornerstone, my bright morning star, I'm coming out." I got goodness and mercy and he is keeping me alive. I am going to make it. I might have to pray all night long, but I know that Jesus heard me. I am coming out of this. I am a survivor.

I cannot give up now. My God shall supply my every need.

Distraction 101

In a season of life where things are supposed to be upbeat and positive, it was difficult to maintain a positive attitude. Even though problems, challenges, and crises are a part of everyday life, I just did not want to think you have to deal with anything negative as your retirement comes through. Well, that was my way of thinking, but not as it was going to be during my new season.

This was the time in my life that I was supposed to be "freer" than I had been in years. My retirement was near. My son, Regis, was engaged to a lovely young lady, Samantha. Also, several trips were on my agenda. Traveling is just one of the things that I really liked to do. Ahead of me was a list of pleasurable activities, including retirement parties, dinners, bridal showers, and the pleasure of meeting Regis' new-in-laws. The dreary winter days were gone. There were no family emergencies. I was just feeling so blessed and not stressed about anything. Anticipation was not going to get the best of me.

How quickly things changed. In March of 2002, while taking an early morning shower, I thought that I felt a lump in my right breast. For a moment, I could not believe what I had felt. Completing my shower and other morning rituals, I attempted to complete my normal day. This did not happen. Beneath the surface and my composed look, fear was lurking, but I refused to acknowledge it. Finally, the day came to an end. It was difficult to not think about my discovery; therefore, I decided to conduct a breast test of my own.

While completing my examination, I again felt the lump. Feeling frightened and not so sure of myself, tears began to flow. Silently, I realized that God's grace was needed at this time. Silently, I asked God to guide me through this situation. I finally dressed myself and just sat down on my bed.

Attempting not to think about my biggest fear, I asked myself where do I start to address my findings? In the past, I have found real comfort turning to God in prayer. When giving my fearful circumstances to God, I took comfort in his words, "Be strong and courageous," for it is God who is underneath the surface of things and behind the scene to make things better.

Retreating to questioning God, I could not understand this fear that I was experiencing. For the next few months, I was overcome with crying, depression, and fear of the unknown. Questioning what was happening to my body became my private focus. Not being ready to share this secret with anyone, I decided to lighten up on myself and continue to work on my son's pending groom's dinner, plans for my trips to Georgia and to Louisiana. Relaxing and convincing myself that all was well became quite a task. Daily affirmations that my "every need would be met," meditation, and prayer aided in my day-to-day coping and struggle. Physically, I felt fine. Psychologically, I was a wreck. As I asked God to be merciful, and to teach me to remain spiritually calm, the activities were on target.

Wondering where God was in the midst of this mind-boggling event, it became clear that I had asked that same question before. During my father's last days, I found myself becoming angry with God. Crying, I asked how could this be part of any "God-guided design?" Unable to comprehend why "church-going and praying folks" have to face such uncertainty, I began to lose sleep—another problem for me. My family and friends used to say that "I could sleep anywhere, anytime, through anything, and even on a picket fence." They noticed that I had become more impatient and rather irritable, as well as noticeably frustrated. Some friends and family attributed this to the pending family visits and the groom's dinner. So I just allowed them to continue believing this scenario.

Fortunately, I received a wake-up call. During one of my inspirational readings, I realized that my way of thinking and method of dealing with this situation were out of whack. Somewhere I had heard that learning to accept God's will was a part of the master plan. Also, that getting out of this world includes some pain and problems, if God's plan was believable. The time had come for me to let go of this pity party and tap in to my faith. It was time to learn how my spiritual belief could help me to understand and accept my physical and mental challenges.

According to the teaching of Silent Unity, a bridge carries a roadway over what seems like an impassable obstacle. Well, prayer is a kind of a bridge which affirms words and healing in every cell of the body. Closing my eyes, I imagined that the lump that I had felt in my breast was opening and responding to healing. I believed that the words of my faith were charged with spiritual energy, and that they had the power to generate healing. Struggling with my personal issues, I began to pray excessively. I remembered some of my favorite verses, such as "ask in faith, never doubting..." (John 1:6). Hebrews 11.1 states "faith is the substance of things hoped for." Hosea 4:6 says "my people are destroyed for their lack of faith."

Struggling to face reality and my choices, I still had not decided to share my findings with anyone. Mediating and reading my *Daily Word, Science of the Mind,* and praying the rosary, I reached a turning point and a shift in thinking. Rewind and replay. Never had the God I know and love ever failed me. The devil had taken enough of my thoughts, feelings, energy, and time. As John 11:43-44 put it: "Loose ... and let me go." Clearly, I could feel the spirit telling me to move on and make a plan of action. God had given me the green light. He has the answer. His words hold the keys. Now is my time and the season is now to find out that God's words revive and make things possible. I declared the works of God in my life (Psalms 118:17). I continued to meditate, saying special novenas to "Our Lady of Lourdes," reinforcing a sense of hoping and a fuller appreciation of life's wonders.

Having worked hard and played hard, whether volunteering, teaching second grade, high school, or college students, mentoring young future teachers, shopping, or just reading a great book, attending mass, reading inspirational books and giving thanks to God for all the blessings in my life, I was afraid of the unknown—and the possibility of having breast cancer was added to that list of unknowns. Every day carried its own trouble and would take care of itself. As found in Matt. 6:34, "Therefore, do not worry about tomorrow, for tomorrow will take care of itself." Through prayers and meditation, I stopped thinking with my head and listened to my heart. Having faith that God provides for all my needs and the directions to accomplish them, I began to lose some of the fear. Because I believed in the Word of God, the time was now to let my faith take over. I reflected on Job 22:21: "Agree with God, and be at peace; in this way, good will come to you," My hope to address my concerns became more of a reality.

I began to mentally prepare to better understand what had been happening to me and to turn my wheels in another direction. Once I started looking after myself better, my thinking seemed to become clearer. Ecclesiastes 1:9 reminded me "What has been, will be again; what has been done, will be done again; there is nothing new under the sun." In Christ, there is hope for every battle and new situation. Rethinking and deciding to go ahead with my plans for the month of April, I contacted Silent Unity and Science of the Mind prayer partners and asked them to pray with me and for me. Praying, they informed me that "the Spirit directs and heals our loves." Strongly believing in the power of prayer to create miracles in my life, my daily tasks and preparations for traveling and my son's groom dinner became very bearable, as well as enjoyable.

Still, I realized that I had not addressed my plan of action. It was time to call my primary-care physician and make an appointment. Not wanting to dampen my spirit, nor disturb my calmness, my secret was still safe with me. After the trips, bridal showers, and celebration, I would inform my family and close friends of my struggle. I wanted to be ready and confident for my "peace of God," which passes all understanding (see Philippians 4:7). Meanwhile, convinced that all things would work out for my good, and despite my physical challenge, life seemed to be great.

Affirming "divine order," I let God do what God does best, and let him bring about the solutions that only he can. Assuring myself that "divine order" was very active in every area of my life, all I needed were healthy strategies to support what I needed to get done. Burying myself in the projects, I couldn't linger much longer. I called my primary care physician and scheduled an appointment. Finally, with creative planning, and help from Prince's song, "We are not afraid to play in the sunshine," the sun was shining. Spring house cleaning was in full swing. The trip to Louisiana was enjoyable. The bridal shower was fantastic. The wedding celebration was on target. Both joy and sadness were a part of my life. It was time to position myself, declare the revelations, and remains strong for God's continuing favor and blessings. He is a God of incredible details and unexpected favors.

During those months, I did learn a lot about myself. First, I could keep a secret. Secondly, I was mentally and physically stronger than I thought. Third, realizing how much energy and strategies I had to master to appear happy, fulfilled and without worry, I could win an Academy Award. Actively engaged in perfecting this persona, the possibility of what I might be facing was never out of my mind. In the human experience, being a "multi-tasker" is quite common. Seemingly, I was engaged in handling a variety of situations at one time and was good at all of them. Nonetheless, keeping this secret was harder than giving childbirth or having dental work performed.

The month of May had finally arrived and was quickly moving on. This reminded me of the festivities that were growing closer. The end of my secret was ever so close. The guests were arriving. My brother, Preston, sister Deborah, cousin Judie, and Regis' in-laws had traveled from California, Virginia, and Georgia. All just wanted to unwind and get comfortable. Judie and I decided to work on some decoration and seating arrangements. As I was reminiscing and catching up on the latest family news, for some unknown reason, I began to tell her about my findings. Why had I done this? Really. I had no idea. The words just tumbled out. At long last, the secret was out.

Not interfering with my story, Judie listened attentively. When I finally stopped talking, she asked, "Have you been to see your doctor?" Of course, my response was, "No, I have not." Also, I informed her that I had not shared this with anyone else. Informing me that the secret was mine to share, she stated that she would pray that I would feel up to sharing with the rest of our family. I told her that I did have an action plan, which was to unfold as soon as this celebration was over. She thanked me for feeling free enough to share this with her, and asked what she could do to help me now. I thanked her for listening, not passing judgment, and asked that she remember me in her prayers. Breathing seemed to be easier. It was bedtime. The feeling was great. Fear of the unknown was still there, but for the moment, it was moved to the back burner.

According to the psychiatrist, Judith Orloff, negative energy can come from thoughts, feelings of fear, and anger. Also, she tells us that positive energy comes from holding thoughts of hope, compassion, forgiveness, and faith in knowing that we can connect to the divine. The next morning, I felt it was time to share my pressing situation with my brother and sister. My sister, the nurse, using her professional voice, explained that I should not jump to conclusions, but should seek medical advice. My intellectual brother concluded that in order for me to consider making a useful action plan, seeking medical opinions was necessary. They were both shocked that I thought it was best to harbor this secret for so long. They had me agree that two things had to be done. First, I needed to share my findings with my children, Regis and Samantha. Secondly, I had to keep my appointments and follow the doctor's recommendations. I thanked them for their support, and we said a prayer in agreement. Jesus said, "If two of you agree on Earth concerning anything you ask, it will be done for you by my Father in heaven" (Matthew18:19). Judie, hugging me, told me how proud she was of me. Joking, they all said that I was finally growing up . One of the family's jokes was that I was afraid of sickness. Now I was demonstrating that I had gotten over my fears.

Finally, the big event was over. A good time was had by all. It was time for friends and family to depart. Spring was gone. It seemed that summer came and exited just as quickly. Mentally preparing myself, looking at my action plan again, I knew that it was time to move. One article that I had read summed it all up for me. In a nutshell, it said: "God has created me for a life of health and abundance." Continuing to turn to God for wisdom and guidance, I reminded him that my family needed me, my son needed me, and he needed me too. During the morning, noon, and night, pleading my unknown case with Jesus and his mother, Mary, I asked them to intercede on my behalf. God teaches that "we can choose life or death." I did not want to die. I wanted to live and declare his works. (See Psalms 118:17.) I had many tasks to complete and many chores to finish. I asked God to be patient with me. He revealed to me that he had not brought me this far to be crushed by illness.

Juila Cameron writes, "Allowing for improvement while not expecting perfection, I am an open work in progress." I thanked God for another day and warm family. The words of *The Science of Mind teachs:* "Nature demands the change in order that we may advance my spiritual practices, and internal fortitude. I was experiencing joy and a physical high as I moved through my distractions."

Faith in God increased as I remembered that "Yesterday is gone and tomorrow may never come." Matthew 6:34 states, "Therefore, do not worry about tomorrow, for tomorrow will take care of itself." Feeling better, with a renewed sense of inner security and believing in the direction that God would take me, my stress was dramatically reduced.

More happiness flowed into my life with a combination of more restful sleep and higher levels of functioning. Trusting God even when I did not know what was going on with my body made me realize that he will give me the strength to "carry on." Like Peter, I declared, "Lord, I do not know where to go, but you have the words of eternal life" (John 6:68). In my life, the Lord was moving in all kinds of ways.

Mary, my sister and friend, reminded me that time was not my friend. First, it was neccessary for me to contact my primary-care doctor. Therefore, I scheduled an appointment and kept it. This was not as hard as I had imagined. Upon completing the physical examination during which she asked several pertinent questions, the doctor acknowledged a lump in my right breast too. Her recommendation was to have a mammogram. Inquiring when my last mammogram was taken, she was shocked to learn that at my age, I had never taken one. I explained that for many personal reasons (and that I was just a plain coward), I had elected not to follow the recommended mammogram.

After she suggested that I consider having one done now, the referral papers were written. On the way home, I asked God for a new grace as I come to terms with my next step. I thought of a line of scripture: "Lift up your eyes and see your own neediness and allow me to help you." This allowed me to drive without anxiety. Now I had to take responsibility. I realized that grace is always sufficient to take me where I needed to be. Imploring him to open every door and lift up all the covers that have been placed on my health, I needed to have all hidden things removed.

For the first time, it was necessary to address my newly found, real fears. I called my son, family, Mary, Bea and I informed them of the day's developments. Knowing how I felt about having mammograms done, they were relieved that I had agreed to follow the doctor's recommendation. Feeling better about the situation and thanking God for such supportive friends and family, I called the clinic. Scheduling an appointment as early as possible was the goal. My appointment was made for 8:30 AM on Monday. Fear—attempting to raise its ugly head—caused me to become frighten again. Having heard so many horrible mammogram stories, I prayed that God would remove this feeling and allow me to only think about what I needed to do. On a three-way call to Mary, Bea, and Regis, I informed them of my pending examination. After giving a word-by-word description of my conversation with Mary and Regis, Bea informed me that she would take off from work and drive me to take the test. I thanked Bea, and gladly accepted her offer. We prayed that God would bless all of as he brought us to new places of hope. We ended our conversation.

Before I knew it, it seemed that the weekend was over. Monday was here. Because I rose earlier than usual, I had time to complete my morning meditation and then get ready to keep this appointment. Driving to Bea's home, I asked God for his traveling grace and mercy. Continuing and asking for strength to obey whatever outcome of this test the Holy Spirit would see fit, I finally arrived at Bea's home. Changing cars, Bea took over. As we melted into the early flow of the Bishop Ford Freeway's traffic, Bea noticed that I was not as talkative as usual. She suggested that we should agree in prayer to give this situation to God because He is in charge—not us. So we prayed, "Lord, anoint my heart and eyes so as to hear and look at this situation from his side." This was quite helpful. My pulse was beating faster. My heart seemed to be pounding out of control, but I was cool. One way or another, I realized that my life would never be the same.

Ongoing Developments

I wish that I could say that I continued to feel like the improved "big girl."

No, I felt like I was at my first scary job interview. I had a promise to keep. As I completed the necessary paperwork, waiting became my enemy. As anyone who knows me would tell you, I am not the most patient person. Taking out some of the reading material that I had brought along, I attempted to read, but the concentration was not there. Finally, my name was called. In the examination room, the technician explained the procedures as she demonstrated what would be taking place. The more she continued to explain the procedure, the more I thought, "What am I doing here?" With tears streaming down my face, facing the young lady, I said, "I will have to reschedule."

At first, she was quiet, then, she softly asked, "Do you believe in that cross that you are wearing?"

Surprised at her questioning, I responded, "Yes, I do."

"Well," she stated, in a matter-of-fact tone, "you must know that you are not alone!"

Finding my voice and feeling somewhat embarrassed, I confirmed that I am a believer of the crucified and in the power of his word. I thanked her for her patience and professional help. I agreed to allow her to start and complete the examination. Next, I had to have an ultrasound and a sonogram. Not being as frightened of these, I was not prepared for the pains that were involved. Those hurt more than the mammogram.

Finally, I was told the examinations were over. She instructed me to get dressed and return to the waiting area. They gave me a clearance and informed me that the results would be sent to my primary-care doctor. Bea and I headed back to the south suburbs: home. Upon arrival at Bea's home, I retrieved my car and headed home. I was so relieved that I had successfully completed this task without fainting. I could not wait to call my friends , family and share my experiences. Everyone was so surprised that the day had gone quite well for me, despite the small discomforts that I had experienced. In a quiet moment of reflection, I felt a stirring of divine inspiration. Giving thanks for whichever path I will have to take, it was time to step forth and prepare for the evening. Not knowing what adventures were in store for me, I was listening for the small voice of God within my heart that would allow me to step forth in confidence and trust.

> *"Teach me your way, O Lord that, I may walk in your truth. Give my undivided heart to revere your name."*
> (Psalms 86:11)

I quieted my thoughts, and decided to release my thoughts to God. Without warning, my evening was coming to an end. Letting go of how things should be and trusting that "thy will be done," I turned my thoughts off and prepared dinner. There was a need to fight off negative thoughts or anything that might upset my train of thinking. Tomorrow would bring its own brand of circumstances and/or opportunities. At this very moment, I just wanted to bathe, rest, and not be weary. Human nature being what it was, I was attempting to remain as positive as possible. This was a promise that I had made to myself as well as my family and friends.

Positive thinking kept me going for the next couple of days, and then the dreaded call from my primary doctor came. She informed me that it was necessary for me to go to her office. At this time, physically, I had not experienced any pain; therefore, I felt fine. Eating healthier, drinking more water and green tea, getting more rest, I was taking better care of myself. Being of the mindset that all was well, I dressed myself and called Mary to inform her of the doctor's call. She asked if I wanted her to meet me there. I thanked her and said that wouldn't be necessary. I told Mary that I would call her upon my return. With that I was out the door. I had business.

As I drove to the doctor's office, I said my rosary. I reminded myself that loving God does not mean you will not get sick or have problems. Sometimes, God uses sickness to discipline us. He takes us through difficult times and storms. Therefore, whatever the results, he can trust me not to fall out, kill myself, give up, or stop praying and praising his name. The results of the mammogram, ultrasound, and sonogram indicated that I had breast cancer. By these words, I was astounded. At first, I just looked at the doctor. Up to this point in my life, my only illnesses had included tonsil removal, gallstone surgery, sinus headache, toothache, childbirth, and few minor injuries. After I regained my composure and found my voice, I inquired about my next step. Eye examinations, dental, and partial yearly examinations were my choice of medical examinations. Thus far, I had been rather healthy. Listening quietly to her medical opinions and recommendations, I began to wonder, why me? Why this time in my life? In my heart of hearts, despite the uncomfortable feeling, I knew it was silly for me to be second-guessing God, but still, I did. The old saying that you will not leave this world without some major pains and/or problems revisited my memory. "OK, Marva," I told myself, "you have enjoyed this pity party long enough. Now it is time to let go and let God."

Taking conscious control of my thoughts and feelings, I realized that there is not a reason for me to not believe it when the Bible says that God directs my steps. God's words are full of power. Earlier, in the Science of Mind,I had read that "the difference between life and life situation is that my life never needs to be healed, only my life situations."

Coming to terms with my new situation, it was time to focus and allow God to open the doors to my solutions, despite the battle. My brother, Preston, during one of our many conversations, jokingly told me to "stop fussing and listen to what God was saying to me." The conference had come to an end. It was time for me to make some tough decisions.

Even though the pain was great, I felt relieved to know. Not feeling as frazzled as I had anticipated, I allowed myself to surrender to the "power and presence of God within me." My drive home was not frustrating. Telephoning Mary, I related my discovery. In her own, quiet way, Mary asked what she could do to help me work this out.

She reminded me that this was the holiday season. She suggested that we revisit my action plan. Agreeing with her, I gave the names of the surgeons and hospitals that the doctor had shared with me. If it was at all possible, I wanted to get this done before Christmas. Why before Christmas? Really, I have no rhyme or reason, but this did give me a point of focus. With all it entails, Thanksgiving was fast approaching. Therefore, there was not much time to fool around.

Mary decided to come over to my home. Sitting in the kitchen, she started making telephone calls. After studying the list, we decided that we would make an appointment to see whichever surgeon had an opening. This was a crazy way to select a surgeon. Since we did not know any of them anyway we reasoned that this method could not be that negative. Brilliant! Addressing the problem motivated me to get on with this situation. It removed some of the fear and negativity I had felt earlier. Thanking God for Mary and her nurturing, we had a cup of coffee and focused on our journey. The power of preference, focus, and motivation to address the barriers that were limiting my life became reinforced. Letting go of the negative feelings; being scared was not going to steal my blessings. Another one of my favorite verses at this time was "...in all your ways, acknowledge him and he will make straight your paths." (See Proverbs 3:6.) At that moment, I was trusting God to guide me and not to allow any moments from my past to cloud my vision.

Each call brought questions about what was the best action to take. How wonderful it was to know that I was not alone in making the simplest to the most complex decision. At last, Mary had made contact with a surgeon who had an opening. He was located at Ingles Hospital, in Harvey, Illinois. According to advertisements, this hospital was reported to have a "top-notch" cancer hospital in the city. It was rather close to my location. Another of my sisters in Christ, Mae, offered to drive me to this appointment. I accepted her offer. My son and the Cades would meet us at Ingles Professional Building. Upon arriving at the hospital, I registered and waited to be seen by the doctor. Relief overtook my anxiety. Before long, Regis and the Cades arrived. Then, I was called into the examination room.

The assisting nurse was very cordial and professional. The surgeon was not to my liking or very professional. He seemed to be in a big hurry and had no time to listen to my concerns. I had picked up a copy of my films, as instructed by the receptionist. He did not even look at my films. He said that I needed a mastectomy. Inquiring why could he made such a recommendation without opening my films and looking at them, he apologized and opened the films. Addressing me, he informed me that I might need another biopsy. He advised me that I probably could not have reconstruction the same day. Because I was not feeling very satisfied, I just wanted out of his office. I dressed as quickly as I could, and headed out to my family and friends. They could see that I was quite disturbed. I explained what had transpired. They understood why I was so perturbed. Thanking Regis and the Cades, Mae and I decided to stop for lunch.

Returning to my home and thanking Mae for her friendship, I headed to the telephone to give Mary a call. She came right over. Taking out the list, Mary began making calls again. After several calls, Mary located a surgeon who had an appointment available. She made an appointment for that Thursday morning of the same week. Believing that no condition was incurable or irresolvable, the need to locate a surgeon was now more apparent and urgent. It has been established that, "for God, all things are possible." Backed by faith, conviction, and affirming in prayer, I trusted in the power and glory of the Lord with all my heart. (See Proverbs 3:5.)

Each day briought questions concerning the best actions to take. How wonderful it was for me to realize that I was never alone when making the simplest to the most complex decision. On Thursday, I was up early. Refreshed by sleep, I was ready to get the show on the road. As I drove to Mary's home, I prayed that God's grace would support me and help me to align myself with his compassion and mercy. Finally, arriving at Mary's, we switched cars and moved into the flow of Chicago's massive early-morning traffic. From the beginning of this visit, I witnessed in the face of the receptionist such a pleasant and warm soul. I sensed this was *the one*. The surgeon was "seasoned," professional, and caring. After reviewing my films and test results, he explained that located in my right breast were two different types of cancerous tumors, which was really uncommon.

Recognizing that I was very frightened, the doctor explained why he thought I would benefit from a radical mastectomy. Feeling nervous and numb, I asked the doctor how many surgeries of this type had he performed. This seemed to tickle him. Looking at me, he said, "That does not matter if I am not successful with yours." On that, we did agree. Discussing what I needed and what I wanted led to the question of breast reconstruction possibly on the same day as the surgery. He suggested that I discuss with options with my family. Also, he advised that if I was serious about the reconstruction, I should seek an appointment with the plastic surgeon. In closing, I asked if it would be possible to have this done before the Christmas holidays. He responded that this would be possible. He added that I should contact the plastic surgeon as soon as possible, because they needed to discuss possible surgery dates.

Jokingly, on the way home, I said to Mary, "If Northwestern Memorial Hospital is good enough for the mayor of Chicago's wife and all other dignitaries, it is good enough for me." In spite of the diagnosis, I had a good feeling about my circumstances. With all my heart, I trusted in the power and glory of God. "Trust in the Lord with all your heart" (Proverbs 3:5). Divine order was opening the door for me. We arrived at Mary's home. I thanked her for always being there, and I headed home. I gave myself time for a little nourishment. I decided to take a breather. A couple of hours later, I telephoned Regis and Samantha and shared my diagnosis with them. I decided that a good, hot soak would feel great. I prepared my soapy bath. A few minutes later, Regis called to ask how I was really holding up. He said that I did sound fine, but it seemed that something was still unsettled. I told him that the possibility of having reconstruction was still very much on my mind. In his own quiet way, he said, "Mom, you will already be out, so plan to have it done, too. You know if you don't, you will not go back later." I had not thought of it in that way, but what he shared was so true. I said that I would think about it, and that it was now prayer time.

This had been a rather long day, but it was still not over. I called my brother, sister, and extended family, and repeated my day's adventure. Everyone agreed with Regis. I should consider having both surgeries on one day, if that was possible. I thanked them for their opinions, love, concerns, and promised to follow through on making the appointments. I got back to Mary, and informed her of my various conversations, as well as my decision to have both surgeries done on the same day. She told me she was happy that I had reached this decision. The very next day, we sought an appointment with the plastic surgeon. Now, it was time to have a light meal and just relax. Bedtime was not far off.

As I communed with the Holy Spirit, an inner experience of tranquility allowed me to not dwell on my condition. I felt renewed in my awareness, whatever my condition, with support of family and friends. The knowledge that they were each there for me completed my day. Without dwelling on the negative, my inner peace was present with newfound confidence. In reviewing the day's events and thanking God for the many smiling faces of the cheerful and conscientious people who helped to make my day, I felt blessed. I was grateful.

With a different attitude and appreciation for a good night's sleep and an early rise, I was ready to face all that this day had to offer. Per our previous conversation, Mary came over to call the plastic surgeon's office to make an appointment. I made a pot of coffee, ate a hearty breakfast and awaited her arrival. Joanne Blum wrote, "When we are up against our edges, uncomfortable, or confused, chances are good we are also on the threshold of spiritual discovery." For the first time, I really began to realize that my life—as I knew it—was about to change. This would be a major turning point in my life. I had to trust in God. I had to believe and surrender, and not interfere with the solutions to what once were my problems. My task now was to refrain from worrying. I had to trust in God, and believe, surrender, and know that God would answer my prayers.

The doctor had an open appointment. On the following Monday, at 8:45 AM, I was scheduled to meet the plastic surgeon. Again, as appointments go, this was a pleasant experience. Starting with the receptionist, the intake personnel, and ending with the doctor, everything was done to take away any apprehension that I was experiencing. With vibrancy and clarity, the steps and options were professionally explained to me. Yes, the doctor was available. He would contact the surgeon. They would select a date and time that was suitable—and before the Christmas holidays. Feeling that I was on the right path once again, Mary and I decided to have breakfast. At this time, we would discuss and refine what had just happened.

At times, things may seem chaotic, but underneath, divine order was present and active. Daily Word had an article that stated "Just as the proverbial dark cloud has a silver lining,so every dark midnight has a background glow." Due to all the negativity associated with cancer diagnosis, silently, I was relieved to learn that it was not always a quick death sentence. I informed my family and extended family members in Louisiana, Texas, California, New York, Georgia, South Carolina, Maryland, D.C., and Illinois of my pending surgery. The prayer chains were formed. During my praying, I continued to ask God to help me to walk in faith with him. I also asked that he allow my problems to become his, as we were all in the flow of things.

Confirmation came. December nineteenth had been assigned as the date to have the procedures done. The next nineteen days would be some of the most challenging of my life. One of my dear friends had a saying that seemed appropriate at this time. It simply said "Life is not measured by the breaths you take, but by the moments that take your breath away."

At times, it was hard to remain focused. Some days, I attempted to work on my holiday agenda. Wanting not to leave anything that I could do for others to do, I was busy checking my bed linens, sending out cards, completing my holiday shopping and house cleaning. It was time to pull out decorations. This quote, from an unknown author, inspired me: "Life is like a rainbow: You need both the sun and the rain to make the color appear." Reading this reminded me that I needed my pending surgery to sustain life as well as enrich my life. December nineteenth would give me an opportunity to start new. So attempting to let go of my preconceived notions about cancer, I prayed that God would come into my heart. I promised to be receptive to his will. Not allowing this to dampen my spirit, I attended a few holiday socials with family and friends. Also, going to the library, I checked out some light reading materials.

As December nineteenth was getting closer, the action plan was being revised. The encouraging thing was what it seemed that I had been waiting for and attempting not to be weary about was coming to an end. In some way, the anticipation was being fulfilled . The time had come. While I was busy trying to figure things out, God had already worked it out. All the major players in this situation had planned how this day would unfold. I can remember clearly how things changed in an instant. The exciting thing was that we did not have to shoulder this day's activities alone. The night before, all the telephone calls, prayers, words of encouragement, and prayers made me feel so special and appreciative. My son, daughter-in-law, and my Chicago friends were in charge of the revised plan. The group had decided that it would be best for Mary to pick me up at my home and deliver me to Northwestern Memorial. The rest of my "entourage" would meet us at the hospital.

On December nineteenth, at 5:00 AM, Mary arrived at my home with bag in hand. I prayed about the situation and told God the most important thing to me was my relationship with him. I also asked him to keep my heart and attitude right during this surgery and reconstruction because this would be a very long day. He had given to me the peace that I needed because I had put my hope in him. (See Romans 5:5.)I know I serve a God who knows every human emotion that I experienced. He got tested, tired, mad, and sad through his various journeys; therefore, I gave this to him in prayer.

At 6:00 AM, we arrived at the hospital and approached the admitting desk. Checking in completed, I was advised to have a seat and wait to be called. My family and friends had arrived too. We exchanged greetings and waited for my name to be called. Saying a silent prayer, I asked God to go before the medical team and watch over each of us this day. I realized that it was not Mary's faith, Father John's faith, my family or my friends' faith, but my faith that I had to rely on this day. This was truly between my God and me. As far as I am concerned, December nineteenth is my new birthday. That was the day the things God had spoken to me in my spirit would become a reality. I have never been quite the same since.

Let me explain it this way: The admittance person came and introduced herself to all of us. For such an early start of the day, all of the people we encountered were friendly, upbeat, and pleasant. This made everything so refreshing. After they explained the important factors of the day, it was time to move to the surgical waiting area. Mary and Mary Ann were allowed to accompany me into that area. I shared my thoughts with my family and friends. We kissed and away we went.

First, I had to change into the surgical garb. Then, the surgical team came and introduced themselves. Finally, the surgeons came and explained again what would be taking place, but first a lymph node biopsy would have to be done. By this time, I really needed to go to the ladies' room. Getting Mary's attention, I expressed my concern. Not realizing that the plastic surgeon had heard our conversation, I was shocked when he responded, "Oh, I will take you. We need to talk anyway." At first, I thought he was joking and so did my friends. Turning toward my friends, he said, "Tell her, 'See you later' Because she will see you later." To the bathroom we went. Mary and Mary Ann returned to the waiting area to join the others.

As he explained the procedures that would be done, the doctor assured me that everything would be fine. He asked if I had any questions or comments. Yes, I had a comment. I explained to him that I did not use my first name (Mary), so he should not attempt to wake me up after surgery by calling me Mary. Instead, I asked that my middle name, Marva, would be used to get my attention. Otherwise, I probably would not respond. He laughed and agreed to share this information with the team. Back to the waiting area we went. Lying down, I was ready to move on. This is all I can recall. Later that night, I woke up in my hospital room, hungry and wondering what time it was.

My son, daughter-in-law, and Mary were all standing at the foot of my bed. The nurse was busy taking my vitals and checking on me. First asking what time it was, I inquired about having something to eat. Those were my first words. Fluffing my pillows, the nursing attendant stated she thought I was asleep. Also, that she would check with the head nurse to see if I could have something liquid and chipped ice. That sounded great to me. I thanked Regis and Samantha for remaining at the hospital all this time. I suggested that they go home and get some much needed rest. It had been a long day for them. They all agreed. As they left, they all said that they would return later in the day.

The early morning of December twentieth proved to be quite difficult. Pain was everywhere. Attempting to reposition my body was even more difficult as well as just a thought. It was harder to find a comfortable position.I buzzed for the nurse, and explained the nature of my call. Right away, she entered and explained the pump that was attached to me and how to use it. It was still early morning, but that did not deter the taking of vitals, and a million questions to be answered as bright lights shined in my face. Now, attempting to return to sleep was a big joke; not a comfortable position was to be had. I was still very hungry. I could not lie on my stomach or right side, and my back was not cooperating. According to Dr. Harvey Chochinov, professor of psychiatry and director of the Manitoba Palliative Care Research Unit, in Winnipeg, Canada, "Problems with sleeping and lack of energy in cancer patients can be assumed to be simply part of the cancer experience." Trust me, this was just the beginning of my sleep-related problems.

Early, around daybreak, the medical team made its appearance. Everyone was very upbeat and pleasant. They explained that the surgery had been successful and everything seemed to be going as planned. They examined me and asked if I had any questions. Of course, food was still on my mind; therefore, I asked if I would be getting a breakfast tray. They promised that my tray would be on the way. They moved out to visit with other patients. The nurse's aide arrived and asked if I wanted my shower. I accepted her offer. Maybe this might make me feel better. After the shower, I asked if it was possible for me to sit up for a while. This proved to work out fine. I sat up and began my meditation. I thanked God for his grace and favor. After I asked him to help me see myself as he had created me, to be "... strong, healthy and whole." My breakfast tray finally arrived. It was all liquid, but filling. My room was cleaned and the bed made. This had been a great morning. Calls from my family and friends, get-well cards, flowers, visits from my children and Mary made this a great day.

Day by day, growing stronger and with good medical reports and fewer pains, I did learn to take slow walks around the nurses' station and the corridor near the rooms. Walking was not as easy as I had anticipated. Those stitches seemed to be in charge of my every movement. Refusing to allow this to deter my steps, I concentrated on the beautiful Chicago skyline to distract me from my painful steps. Physically, I was feeling great. Christmas was around the corner. I wanted to go home for Christmas. My medical team, family, and friends were very pleased with my progress and positive attitude.

The twenty-third of December proved to be out-of-the-ordinary. For the first time, I did not wish to sit up, take a walk, or do anything. Not being able to explain my actions, I just started to cry. Of course everyone was stunned, including me. Inquiring about my pain level, the medical team decided that maybe I needed to speak to the social worker. Agreeing, I did talk with her, but still could not determine why I was in a state of depression. Perhaps it was renewed fear or just the devil attempting to spook my joy. "OK, Marva, stop with this nonsense!" I thought to myself. "You are so blessed. Take time and count your blessings. You woke up this morning, in your right mind, able to wash your own body, with a caring family, great medical team, tremendous friends, and countless other blessings that you cannot fathom." Feeling ashamed, I turned to the "author of my life" (see Acts 3:15) and prayed that he would pick up and take me to the next level.

As the book of Matthew said, "You have to be ready to do what God wants you to do." I had been taught that suffering and holiness go together. Suffering is a reality, and we cannot escape life. So I told the devil to take a walk. I realized that God was in the business of healing and doing great things. I wanted God to put the "supernatural on my natural." It was time to look at the fact that God was preparing me for something better. The storm clouds in my life were passing. Jesus sent me in the storm to have me come out on the other side. The storm clouds had brewed over my life. He placed me in the storm and did not send me through the "eye of the storm" so I would know that he is the Lord, my God. It was so easy to lose sight of God's power that I had allowed this self-pity to enter my spirit one more time. Getting frustrated is human. This really helped to prove to me that I am still very human.

This spiritual storm woke me up to what I should have been thinking about. I must not allow frustration to take away my success. I thanked God for promoting me so that I could wake up and face my blessings. I was back to planning my departure before Christmas. Aligning my mind with God's will was my first goal. At this time, my second goal was to get home for Christmas. Also, this was the day my cousin, Betty, would arrive and join my recovery team. This wonderful traveling angel left her home in Houston, Texas, to come and see about me. This was unbelievable, but I was ever so appreciative. From various articles about cancer I had read, cancer is a "multi-dimensional disease" and a journey addressing the mind, spirit, and soul. Frustration, exhaustion, and reality led me to believe that I had just experienced my first cancer experience. My attempt to not address what I had just gone through and attempts to remain "normal" and not conform to the "new normal" that I had read about caught up with me. The "new normal" that is life after breast cancer was not as simple as ABC. It was a much more complex situation. Still, I was ready to go home. After all, this was part of the revised action plan.

Finally, December twenty-fifth arrived. The medical team had come in early and approved my discharge. This proved to be a very busy day, as well as a very snowy one. My son and daughter-in-law had come early and had started packing my belongings. The nurse had come and explained the care that I would need before returning for my first doctor's appointment the following week. After I expressed gratitude to all members of the nursing staff, we were on our way home. Despite the cold and snow, it felt good to be on my way home. First, we had to stop at the Walgreen's store and drop off a needed prescription. Once this was done, we were finally at home. My son got me settled in. My daughter-in-law was out the door and on her way to pick up my cousin, Betty. Since none of us had seen each other, I had supplied Betty with a picture of the children, because one of them would be fetching her. On the other hand, for identification, Betty would wear a name plaque in her cap. Again, this was a part of the master plan.

Telephone calls and florist deliveries made the rest of my first day at home exciting. In addition to that, my cat, Ashaa, was very happy to see me. About four hours later, Samantha and Betty arrived safely. For the first time, Betty and I came face to face. Giving her time to freshen up and get settled, we finally sat down to our Christmas dinner. Regis and Samantha had prepared a delicious dinner. Giving thanks to God for his divine gifts of family, friends, children, and all the goods that only he can make visible, we had an enjoyable dinner. Being more at ease, with my circumstance, drainage bottles, soreness, and little weak, I was more aware of not wasting energy on what could not be changed. I was thankful that God had allowed this day to unfold in such a positive way. It was time for Regis and Samantha to depart, go meet some friends, and get some much-needed R & R without worrying about me for a while.

Betty and I sat and talked about family members and her research about our family's history. Catching up on the King Family history, facts that I had not been exposed to or knew about my family was interesting. For several years, she had been conducting and compiling information on my mother's side of the family. This is how she had located me earlier in July of that same year. Betty was very passionate about her research. Also, she was chairperson of the pending King family reunion the following June. For a couple of hours, I seemed to have forgotten about my aches and pains. We discussed whether, God's willing, I would plan to attend this reunion. When I thought about going home, it refreshed me and simply brought to mind the familiar places in Opelousas, Louisiana that I used to call home. Moving back to the present moment, I informed Betty that I needed to call this evening to an end.

Thanking Betty for her presence, it was time to get ready for bed. This would be my first attempt to sleep on my own bed again. Giving thanks to God, and looking back over the last couple of weeks, I remembered that my faith in God's "presence and power" brought peace and quieted my anxiety. Remembering this encouraged me to look to God within for the resources surrounding me. Getting to sleep became a hassle. For some reason, I could not find a comfortable sleeping position. Betty experimented with various techniques, but no luck. Finally, I decided it might be best to sleep in the recliner. Relaxing and doing breathing exercises, I began to relax more deeply and completely.

On the next day, my friend, Bea, came over. She and Betty decided to go to the nearby store and purchase sleep pillows. Also, they decided to talk about my nutrition and compile a grocery list. After they found a pad, we compiled a grocery list. At first, they were not sure that I should be left home alone. After promising them that I would not do anything to harm myself, they left for the stores. Just as they were walking out, one of my dearest friends called to see how I was doing, and to fuss because I had not informed any of my former co-workers about my illness. Explaining that this was my decision, and very soon I would share this experience with her. I thanked her for her understanding and promised to keep in touch with her. It was time to read, pray, and meditate on my blessings. Through daily prayers, which supported me in thinking and living, my thoughts and desires were led by the spirit of God.

After they returned home from the store, Betty and Bea showed that they had been successful. They found two different types of sleeping pillows. After they had prepared lunch, charted my vitals and fluids, it was time for lunch. Betty insisted on preparing a healthy hot meal.

As I waited for the meal, I talked with my siblings in California. I explained how grateful I was for Betty's help, nurturing, and support. My siblings took turns expressing how much they appreciated her coming to see about me. Also, they were thankful that our paths had crossed. Remembering the adage, "God always puts who or what you need in front of you when needed," I realized that Betty's presence made a huge difference in my recovery. Her positive attitude just rubbed off on me.

It seemed that my first week just slipped by so quickly. It was time to make the first of many doctor's appointments. Mary came over to assist Betty. She made the first appointment. Since my arrival, this would be my first time out of the house. In addition to finding something to wear, I was still hooked to the drainage bottles. This did create clothes fitting challenges. After getting it together, we had a great lunch. Betty had prepared my favorite Southern dish—okra gumbo with rice. At good as it smelled, I did not have much of an appetite, but I did attempt to eat a couple of spoons. Betty had such a beautiful spirit. Her presence just made everything so much easier. Without complaining, she took charge of the house, me, errands, and anything that she thought would help me to recuperate more quickly. I seemed to develop all the changes that cancer and its treatments can cause in the sense of taste and smell. From day to day, I experimented with new foods, spices, and fruits. I avoided mouthwash or anything that contained alcohol, so not as to irritate my mouth. I had a better appreciation of things that I was grateful for in my life. Becoming more spiritually aware and appreciative for the positive changes in my life helped me to feel more optimistic for better physical and mental growth. Despite the little physical discomforts, my struggles were not as I had imagined they would be. Thanks be to God.

With hope that each day would be better than the other, I gained great strength. My heart was filled with great hope and a new sense of peace and confidence. Knowing deep within my heart, I had more to experience, learn, do, and enjoy, I anticipated wonderful blessings. Because I found a new sense of divine awareness and a new meaning of opportunities to share, receive and give love, I allowed it to guide my thoughts, words, and actions.

Making a Comeback

According to oncology nurse specialist Ann Culvala of Advocate South Suburban Hospital in Hazelcrest, Illinois, "Survivorship is really the focus of treating cancer." Maintaining a good and positive attitude was Betty's plan of action as well as attack. Each day, she had a schedule of activities, including manicures, pedicures, scrapbooking, facials, and pleasantries. Friends were calling, coming to visit, preparing delicious foods; therefore, my children were relieved of some of the physical pressures associated with caring for an ill family member. Having the hope that my strength would return, despite the pains, night sweats, snowy and frigid weather, my "angels" Mary and Betty were determined to not allow me to get depressed. Daily, I gave thanks for their great care and friendship. Giving thanks for the protecting love of God, I tried to focus on the ways in which I could help myself to get better.

> *"And you will have confidence, because there is hope; you will be protected and take your rest in safety."*
>
> *(See Job 11:18.)*

Since I had selected to not seek a "formal group," the wonderful support that I received from my family as well as those friends I chose to share my "situation" with helped to make each day more bearable. Reading breast cancer-related material, going online to the American Cancer Association on the Web site, and other books that I had selected to read aided my understanding of the "big picture" of breast cancer and its effect on my life. One thing that was quickly pointed out in all of the materials was that "cancer dictated a different lifestyle." I continued to ask God to guide my thoughts and me in his words. It was very important that I not lie in bed all day or sit around having a pity party. My official get-up time was 8 AM. Also, I insisted that my day-to-day hygiene care remained my responsibility. Only if I ran into problems would Betty's help become necessary. Learning to eat breakfast was not as easy. Due to the fact that I was never a lover of eating breakfast and my taste buds were not always cooperating, sometimes it was a battle. For my own good, knowing that I needed to eat a good breakfast, I did attempt to comply.

The weeks were flying by so quickly. Doctors' appointments were kept. The various activities keep my spirit and hope peaceful. Opening my mind and heart to visiting with friends and family, I was grateful for the many ways that I began to experience peace. As I reflected on the weeks that had gone by, I gave thanks for the peace of God that was with me. No matter what I encountered, I took a moment to mentally sort out through experiences of the day just how far I had progressed.

Joy is infectious. Betty's love and joy filled my heart and home. Her uniqueness, personality and individuality allowed me the space and time lo learn to adjust to my recovery and continue to develop my spiritual journey. Betty was the one who suggested and reinforced what I had read about keeping a journal about my breast cancer experience. Mary had instilled in me to keep a journal of medical appointments, medicines, as well as medical questions. Now Betty's idea was added to the mix. As it is written, if you search the Bible to back up your ideas, you will locate a passage:

> *"We are writing these things so that our joy may be complete."*
>
> *(See John 1:4.)*

With great faith and determination, I started to take more responsibility for my daily care. I began to assist Betty with the laundry, breakfast preparations, and shopping. I had to prove that I was self-sufficient. Betty's leave was surely coming to an end. Again, the Cades invited me to continue my recuperation at their home. Expressing appreciation for their friendship and caring, I explained that I still wanted to remain at my home. After conferring with Mary, my children, family, and extended family, a schedule was made. All, if necessary, would be available, and in case of an emergency, one would contact the other. Feeling that I would be fine, I prayed that the right decision had been made. "Let your good spirit lead me on a level path." (See Psalms 143:10.) Feeling spiritually uplifted and encouraged, I released any doubts or fears and gained an attitude filled with hope.

All good things must come to an end. For me, January twenty-third was D-day. Early that morning, Betty departed for home. Counting my blessings and not my trials, with much gratitude, I recognized how blessed I was to have enjoyed Betty's company for nearly a month. With love, faith, and wishes for Betty to enjoy a safe trip home, I tried not to become too emotional. As the evening approached, the telephone began ringing. Friends and family members were checking on me. It would take time for me to get back to living alone. So days and nights did not work out as I had planned, but keeping the faith, I made it. As Silent Unity teaches, "There is always a way to overcome challenges and to achieve success." First, I needed to make daily, detailed plans. Secondly, I had to believe that my family and friends were as near as my telephone. Still, one of my friends insisted on spending nights with me. Not putting up a fuss, I accepted the offer. During the day, the home health nurse would check on my well-being. Family and friends would visit, and prepare or bring huge lunches and/or dinners.

As I began to feel stronger and got my bearings, I realized that my sense of learning and growing in the spirit made my day-to-day healing easier. By speaking to my body and commanding it to come into line with the Word of God, I knew that Jesus had not changed. He is the same yesterday, today, and forever. (See Hebrews 13:8.) He has always been "an encourager and up-lifter" to me. Feeling confident, as well as comfortable, it was an excellent time to see more of the meaning of my life's path and to learn to cope with the challenges that I faced. Something inside of me had nudged me back to reality. I had learned that I had been given the opportunity to uncover my abilities with grace and strength daily. I discovered more about myself during the past month; I was guided by the Spirit's gift. Believing that good awaited me around every "bend in the road," my physical comeback—despite the physical discomforts that I had experienced—helped me to turn the corner. On page 185 of *The Science of the Mind,* it teaches to meditate daily on the "Perfect Life," and daily to embody the "Great Ideal is a royal road to freedom." It was from this place that I learned to find the strength and serenity to face my breast cancer challenges.

All of my family members and friends were very proud of the progress that I was making. Mary, Bea, a host of friends and family members continued to drop in, bringing cooked food, sending cards and flowers, as well as taking me to my many appointments. They all expressed how they saw a new level of maturity and determination to deal with the adverse conditions that had impacted all of our lives. Determined to continue making progress as I moved forward, I affirmed that maintaining my health was now my full-time job. A friend of mine reminded me of the following quotation: "The will of God will never take you where the grace of God will not protect you."

My recovery from reconstructive surgery was on target. The drainage bottles had been removed. The plastic surgeon was very proud of the surgery outcome. Selecting the type of reconstruction that I did meant that I had stomach pains and drainage, too; therefore, walking had not been easy. Otherwise, my healing seemed to be going great. Mentally, I still had issues that caused me to "trip." One day, realizing that this was taking place, I starting silently conversing with myself. (No, I had not lost my mind—just my focus.) Quickly, I regained my composure. Questioning my behavior, I began to challenge my negative thinking. Not allowing the "fog" to clog my memory of how amazing God is and how great he has been to me, I vowed that it was time to get back on track. I faced my demons.

> *For God has not given us the spirit of fear but of power, of love, and of a sound mind.*
>
> *(See Timothy 1:7.)*

Betty continued her weekly telephoning. She encouraged me to take good care of myself. The understanding that God is always with me as a presence of power and caring made my days and nights much better.

I went about my days and nights with confidence, knowing my trust in the "one who never fails me" and the prayers of all my prayer partners all over the world made my recuperation move rapidly. Deciding to stay afloat, I chose from a variety of activities, including work, sleep, rest, and play. Strengthened by the boldness and ease by which my outer circumstances and inner concerns were addresses, I released to God whatever needed to be resolved. Asking him to "Work on me, Lord," I continued to do and to give my best. Without any need to feel that things would not improve, my awareness of God's love and blessings deepened moment by moment.

Rising above the limitations of what I could and could not do, I moved to strengthen my possibilities. I envisioned my recovery as a stepping stone to fulfilling my dreams. I prayed for divine inspirations in fulfilling my dreams of getting back on my feet, and for being healed emotionally, mentally, and physically. It was time to address some complex issues and reach some decisions. It was time to contact the recommended medical professionals to seek their opinions regarding a course of treatment. With my family and Mary, I discussed my decision to move forward and put some closure to this segment of my illness. It was time again to trust in God. He had given me the tools to cope with this challenge; therefore, I trusted in the guidance of his spirit. It was from this place that I found strength to face my first major challenge: the diagnosis of breast cancer. By constantly turning to prayer, I recognized and appreciated the emotional benefits of a more relaxed mind and reduced stress.

Finally, after a year, I contacted Northwestern Memorial Hospital and made an appointment to have a consultation with the oncologist.

The social worker who had been assigned to me was so relieved to hear from me. Members of the follow-up staff would call to check on me, as well as to ask if I had discussed a course of treatment. Of course, my response was no. I was not ready to feel bad or become physically disabled again. They attempted to convince me to "look at the big picture" and to encourage me not to lose sight of the big picture. They would wish me well and encourage me to call if I needed anything.I promised that I would think about it and not throw in the towel, but this was a decision that I had to make. God would help me to work this out, too. As my brother said, "if I would stop and listen, I would hear his answer to my newfound situation."

Facing reality and blowing off distorted thinking, I spent hours on the breast cancer Web sites and in the library, reading all that I could locate on different types of chemotherapy treatments and side effects. I developed a command of the nomenclature needed to communicate with the oncologist. After informing Mary of my decision, she called and made an appointment with the oncologist. As before, she would accompany me to the doctor's office. The routine was the same. Mary would drive us to Northwestern Memorial Hospital. Happy that I had made a liar out of the devil, I felt that a burden had been lifted again. Being a child of God, I was walking in victory.

> *And we know that all things work together for good of them*
> *that love God, to them who are called to his purpose.*
> *(See Romans 8: 28.)*

The first oncologist that we had selected was not taking any new patients. We went back to the list to select another doctor. This time, we were successful. He had an opening available for the following week, so an appointment was made. Another crazy way of doing things, but that is how it happened.

Another door had opened. I now had a new task. Fear, anxiety, and worry were not as strong this time. Holistically, appreciating myself for who I am and how much I wanted to continue progressing, I was drawn to the Sacred Heart Novena League. In a nutshell, it said that "We trust the word of God, hoping all things from his goodness. He made a root flourish beneath the soil and he can make fruitful the darkness in which I find myself." It further explained that the life of God flows through me in "ever-renewing streams of healing energy. Any thought of illness or discomfort was to be released with a new sense of wholeness and peace in my mind and body."

Based on my reading about chemotherapy treatment and what I had heard, this was not an easy experiment. The side effects and treatments were things that I could not get out of my mind. At this junction, I had been feeling great. I was again socializing and my energy level was high. My contacts from Northwestern had continued to reinforce that idea that it was very important that I do all that was necessary to remain healthy. "You have to protect yourself. Taking the recommended treatment will help you to survive longer, remain cancer-free," they declared. Another friend stated, "You have the battle scars; therefore, you must make the right decision." My life might not be the same, but it was still mine.

Using one of the suggestions that I had read, before going for the consultation, I made a list of my concerns. My prayers were to get through the visit. *Help me, Lord!*

I handed Mary my journal, and asked her to record anything of interest that I might need in the future. So began this new journal/notebook. Though it had not made my list, I could feel my mental pressure building, silently. I reminded myself that I had given everything to God in prayer earlier, and that I was safe in his care. As I smiled to myself, I felt better and thought to myself, "Bring it on!" For whatever reason, a new cross to bear was entering my life.

No matter what had occurred before, this was a new day and moment. As they entered the room, the doctor and his assistant introduced themselves to Mary and me. They were very professional as well as pleasant. As he completed his initial examination, the doctor requested that I get dressed and move to consultation suite. Quickly and a little self-conscious, I followed Mary into the suite. They were waiting for us. Once we entered the suite, the doctor started explaining the type of treatment that he thought would be most beneficial for the type of cancers that I had. I had two different cancers in the same breast, which was not a common thing.

Asking if I had any questions, the doctor waited for my response. Tears began to flow. It was like I was having an out-of-body experience. Mary noticed that I seemed not to be breathing. She came over and sat next to me. Consoling me, she inquired about my feelings. I was still not responding. The doctor asked if we needed a few moments alone. Because I was just shaking my head and mumbling no, Mary saw that I needed her to ask the questions. She asked about the type of treatment, and details such as how often they were needed, side effects, and length of treatments. Once all questions had been answered, we thanked them and left. On the way to the parking garage, Mary informed me that she noticed when I had mentally shut down, but she was glad that I seemed to have made a quick recovery. I thanked her for her understanding, friendship, and for always being there; it was time to depart.

On the way home, we decided to stop and have an early lunch. While awaiting our selections, Mary instructed me on the notes that she had taken. She went over my scheduled treatment. As we shared an informative and great conversation, I began to settle down. I thanked

Mary for her patience, thoughtfulness, and kindness and we finished our lunch. Driving back to Mary's home to pick up my car, we discussed the plan of attack for my first chemotherapy session. This time, I needed an additional person to join our team, because the doctor did not want me to drive after completing the treatment. I promised Mary that I would work on this before the date of the session, and we said our good-byes. This had been quite a day! At that point, my little angel whispered into my ear that God was in charge, so why had I allowed the devil to disturb my peace of mind?

Yes, I had allowed the devil to overshadow my thinking again, but he would not get any more attention! Arriving at my home, I thanked God for Mary, the medical team at Northwestern and for giving me loving people in my life. Calling my family and several friends, I shared the information concerning my treatment. They were all very glad to hear my decision to accept the treatment. I explained some of the details which included my worst fear—the possibility of losing my hair—and nausea, joint pains, low red blood cell count, lost of appetite, and the number of treatments. They said they would continue to pray for and with me on this new journey. Also, each offered unconditional support. I stopped to make a cup of tea. I still had a couple of calls to make. Needing to secure someone to drive me back home after my treatments, I contacted one of my oldest childhood friends, Iva, who had offered her service. I explained to her the treatment scenario and how if she was available, she could play a role. We discussed a plan that would allow her to meet us at the hospital. Afterward, she would pick up my car at Mary's and drive me home. Iva said that she was available, so I gave the details that she needed. This was great! The plans were falling into place. Clyde, another friend, would meet us at my home and drive Iva back to the city. Now God had taken care of what I thought was a perplexed situation and produced perfect results. With all of the day's actions, I was ready for a hot bath and a good night's sleep.

According to *Science of the Mind,* "Prayer is what gets me out of the bed in the morning. It is what eases my way down the road. It is the direct line to the power, the presence of God that is in me." Another basic tenet of *Science of the Mind* is "change your thinking, change your life." Talking to myself, I said, "Marva, you can do this." Right here, right now, I was getting back on track. The apostle Paul said,

"Rekindle the gift of God that is within you." (See II Tim. 1:6.) After my morning rituals, I called and scheduled my first of many blood tests. After I informed Mary of the date and time, I decided to take the rest of the day and just enjoy it. Needless to say, the day just flew by. Little did I know that a miracle was taking place. Having had this spiritual awakening, I continued to grow stronger as I learned to face my health challenges. This was my miracle.

The following Monday, at 6 AM, Regis drove to Mary's house. At 6:45 AM, we arrived at the twenty-first floor of Northwestern Memorial Hospital for my blood work. After several attempts to draw blood, the technician said that she needed to get the head nurse. "Oh, what is going wrong now?" I asked myself silently. Also, I knew that I was not going to allow anyone to continue sticking me to get blood. The head nurse came in and informed me that my veins were very small and not cooperating.

Another procedure was being considered. I suggested that if my veins would be accessed for each treatment, it might be best if I could have a port implant. After explaining the importance of the implant, and the fact that this would eliminate the sticking each time I needed a blood count and on days that I would be taking treatment. We decided that this would be the best for all concerned; a date and time were scheduled to have this procedure done. Five days later, my son, Regis, Mary, and I entered Northwestern. It was time for me to have the implant procedure. Praying softly that the presence of God would be with the doctor and staff as they prepared to do this surgery, I was swiftly led to another section of the building for same-day surgery. Joking with the technician, I said, "I hope you know what you are doing." Stopping and looking at me, he said, "I am God's child; therefore, everything is in Divine Order." This was great. Feeling the Spirit was guiding everyone, I said "Thank you, God, for answered prayers." With my thoughts centered in the healing presence of God, I fell asleep. I woke up, a couple of hours later, in another location; my vitals were checked, lunch was served, and I was checked again. The nurse reported that everything was on target. I was given my medical information, and I was discharged. After dropping Mary off at home, Regis took me home. After seeing that I was fine, he headed home.

This began an unbelievable adventure. In amazement, as I recuperated at home and was set to have my first chemotherapy treatment. My journey of wholeness was becoming a reality. Again, this was an early-morning appointment. Mary and I had decided the earlier, the better. This way, we would miss some of the busy Chicago traffic. Iva would join us later. First, I had to go to the lab and get the port activated. Secondly, blood had to be drawn and sent to the laboratory. The wait-and-see began. If the blood count was not good, then there would be no treatment. With my thoughts centered on "let this happen," I sat and waited for the results. Finally, the word came that the pharmacy was in the process of preparing the therapy solution. After giving me a cup of ice and juice, and final instructions, the nurse made final preparation for my first chemotherapy treatment. With my reading materials, journal, puzzle book, and Mary at my side, we watched as the medicine entered my body.

Even though it was a relief to learn that my blood count allowed me to take the treatment, my mind was still in a questioning mode. Rather than allowing Satan to enter my space, I decided to read a booklet entitled "Discovering Series" from RBC Ministries. This series discussed what we should think when sickness or suffering attacks us or someone close to us. What should we do? These inspirational readings helped me to uncover biblical certainties that illustrated how "every child of God can count on him in times of sickness and suffering" using the biblical illustrations, many accounts of several illness, intense suffering, deep sorrow, and untimely deaths. Here are two examples of the illustration:

Miriam (E x. 15:20; Num.12; 26-59)
- **Identify _____ sister of Moses and Aaron**
- **Affliction ___ leprosy**
- **Source ___ God**
- **Reason ___ chastening for rebellion**
- **Result _____ repentance, healing, restoration**
- **Lesson _____ God sometimes uses suffering to chasten his disobedient children.**

Mephibosheth (2 Sam, 4:4:9)
- Identify ____ son of Jonathan, grandson of Saul
- Affliction ____ crippled through a fall
- Source ____ not given
- Reason ____ not given
- Result ____ lifetime affliction with no cure provided
- Lesson ____ God does not always tell us the reason for our suffering.

My treatment was coming to an end. It lasted a little over three hours. During the treatment, I ate the chipped ice so that my mouth would not get sore. Talking with Mary, journaling, reading, and taking a short nap were the activities that I engaged in during this therapy. As she explained my results and the next scheduled treatment, the nurse had me sign a release form. I got dressed and thanked Mary for sitting with me through this ordeal. It was time to head home. As we entered the outer area, we saw Iva waiting for us. I thanked Jesus for providing me with such caring and great friends. Then we headed to Mary's so that we could carry out the plan that we had devised. Once we arrived at Mary's home, Iva and I changed cars. We were headed to the last leg of this adventure. First, we stopped and picked up a couple of items to add to our lunch. Once we arrived at my home, Iva completed our lunch. By this time, Clyde had arrived to drive Iva home. As we shared a great laugh, we all declared that harmony was all around us. In the smallest details of my hours and in the large events of this day, God's guidance led all of us. The resources and the array of opportunities that had been made available today proved to me, more than ever, that God's guidance is always with me. Giving thanks to God for his intercessions, I was ready to just sit and relax for a couple of hours and enjoy my private space.

My second treatment was quite an event. Arriving for my scheduled appointment, I was informed that a new technician would be in charge of accessing my port. Well, as things go, on her first attempt, she was not successful. After I calmed down and focused (finally), I suggested that she contact Jennifer, who had been successful in accessing the port. At first, she wanted to continue on her trial and error, but once I informed her that this was the reason that the port had been implanted—so that I would not have to endure multiple trial-and-error sessions—she reluctantly contacted Jennifer, who worked her magic. The blood was drawn and sent to the lab. The blood count was good; therefore, the pharmacy was instructed to mix the therapy medicine. After they provided me with a cup of chipped ice and a cup of cranberry juice, I was ready to accept my second chemotherapy treatment. With reading materials, meditation material, and prayers to Saint Michael of the Saints, Trinitarian mystic and cancer patron, and Saint Peregrine, patron of cancer victims, and my copy of *Every Day Is a Gift*, meditations for every day which are taken from the Bible and writing of saints all at my side, I settled in for my body to accept this medicine. As I asked God to never allow me to lose my "zest" for life and my appreciation of all that his blessings have allowed me to endure, I gave thanks for being loved and cared for by my Mary, medical staff, many friends and family.

Before I was allowed to go home, I was informed that it would be necessary for me to get a shot of Neupogen in between my treatments. This was to be done daily. On one of his visits, my home care nurse, Bob asked if I would like to learn how to give myself this shot.

Quickly, I responded, "No."

Then he asked if I had a friend he could train to administer this daily shot.

Again, I replied, "No."

My friend, Bea, who was present at the time, said, "I would be willing to learn, that is if she does not mind."

Of course, I asked Bea if she was aware that this had to be done daily, between each treatment. She said that she was up to the challenge. We agreed that she would take the training. Bob began his instructions. And the rest is history! For the next couple of weeks, Bea came each morning and gave me the shot. One of the many side effects of this shot was joint pain. According to research, only 33 percent of patients suffered the side effects. (Guess who fell into this category?) I was so unfortunate to join this elite group of survivors. Since I had not experienced the gum swelling, nausea, or other side effects of chemotherapy, I was a little surprised, but I survived the ordeal.

Stephanie, the social worker, called to check on my well-being and to find out if I had any concerns. My nurse, Jennifer, would also call to check on me. Mary called to remind me that I should be more selective in my food choices. That included that I should not eat tomatoes or tomato-based dishes, gravies, or fried foods. She encouraged me to eat more fresh foods, as well as more fruit. She had been to the grocery store and shopped for items that she thought would help my system. She told me that she was on her way.

As I took deep breaths, I was so grateful that God had blessed me with people, activities, friends and family who filled my heart with the joy of thanksgiving. This experience had helped me to really grow in many ways, as well as spiritually. My friends and family continued to be very supportive. They were amazed at how great I seemed to be doing. So far, I not had experienced chronic insomnia, chills and fever, depression, or hair loss, even though these are common side effects associated with the chemotherapy. Feeling that I had been spared these horrible side effects, my hopes and dreams were being fulfilled.

At the end of my fourth treatment, my hair had not fallen out, my joints were not aching as much, and my appetite was better. Someone I care about deeply asked me a question that caused me to take notice of my hair. Yes, I did notice that my hair looked and felt thinner, but I had plenty of hair. During the change of seasons, my hair did have a tendency to fall out. But in the following days, I did notice longer strands seemed to be left in my brush as I brushed my hair. I called my beautician and shared my concerns with her. She recommended that I come in for a consultation. Immediately, I got myself ready and met her at the salon.

After examining my hair, we agreed that cutting the hair might help soften the blow if and when my hair would fall out. As Liz, my beautician, began the trimming and cutting process, several of the clients could not believe that I was having this done. I attempted not to allow their comments to bother me. I just prayed to maintain a degree of calmness and confidence. The reality is that I was not prepared for this, but I knew that this was my best course of action. Liz continued with the clipping, shaping, and cutting, and then it was time to move to the shampoo bowl. Here, the shampoo person, Jen would take over. Liz would continue once this process was completed.

At the shampoo bowl, everything seemed to be going as it should be; shampooing, conditioning, and jovial conversation. Out of nowhere, I heard this shrilling scream. Just that fast, all of my hair was gone! When Jen towel dried my hair, it stayed in the towel. My head was as bare as a baby's behind. I advised Jen that she had not done anything wrong. It was time to get Liz in on the crisis. I explained to Jen that I had been taking chemotherapy, and that hair loss was one of the side effects. We tried to assure her that all was fine. There was not a dry eye in the shop. Everyone was concerned about my emotional and physical well-being. My response to everyone surprised me. I simply thanked them for their concern and informed them that I been in some ways preparing for this seemingly impromptu moment. Liz made certain that she had done all that she could to make sure that I would not catch cold. As I placed my hat on my now-bald head, I thanked Liz, Jen and all of the other clients for their understanding and sympathy. And I headed for home. I promised Liz that I would call her as soon as I arrived at my home. On my way home, I realized that I was rather composed and doing quite well, despite my present situation.

Talking about another long ride home, this was my third longest one. First was the one after my cancer diagnosis. Second was the ride home after the surgery and reconstruction. Now this one would join that list; the drive home after the loss of my entire head of hair. Even though the doctor had explained that this would probably happen, I really did not believe him. I had heard, from several women who were friends, that some of my friends did not lose their hair. So I had been hoping that I would fall in this category. Reality is a hard pill to swallow. One of my worst fears had come true. Silently, I began to say aloud the "Serenity Prayer" of St. Francis de Sales. It went like this:

> *God grant me the serenity to accept the things I cannot change,*
> *the courage to change the things I can,*
> *and the wisdom to know the difference.*

As I gave voice to my faith, I began to feel better and stronger. With a couple of challenges under my belt, I refused to allow negative energy to enter my space. I placed a copy of Donnie McClurkin's CD medley, *Come This Far by Faith, I Will Trust in the Lord,* and *I Love to Praise His Name,* in my car's CD player; my drive home was inspiring. It helped me to keep from going to a dark place. These songs touched my heart, mind, and soul. Change was scary, but God put me here for a reason, hair or no hair. As soon, as I entered the house, I put on water for a cup of hot tea. It was time to call everyone and inform them of my latest happening.

Telephoning my son and daughter-in-law, Mary, Mrs. Mathis, and Bea, I shared with them my latest incident. As I described how the event unfolded, and the experience's impact on me, each one was surprised that I seemed quite calm and in control. Convincing them that I was fine and not in a state of shock was sort of hard. They asked in one way or another how I remained so much in control. Laughing, I said something to this effect: "Now, I will be able to have any color hair that I want! I can have different-color wigs." Later in the evening, I called my sister and brother, and shared with them the latest episode in my adventure as a breast cancer survivor. Expressing their concern, they wanted to know what they could do. Asking how I was doing, they were surprised that I sounded so positive and was in a joking mood. All of the persons I had spoken to are Southern-born. They knew how important and significant hair was to Southern women, and in their lives. This truly is a story for another time. By this time, I was exhausted and needed some down time. Knowing that my family and friends needed to be made aware of the situation, I also knew that I would be getting a telephone call. Tomorrow was another day. It would bring its own set of concerns and problems. Then I would have to answer the inquiring telephone calls and assure everyone that I was really doing great. After a nice, hot shower, it was time for my dinner and a good night's sleep. I thanked God for his blessings, and went to bed feeling relieved.

From a deep sleep, a loud telephone ringing jarred me. It was a call from my cousin, Judie; the grapevine was working. She apologized for the lateness and for waking me, but she wanted to know how I was coping. I explained to her that I felt fine and was not overwhelmed. I looked at the clock. To my surprise, it was still the same day—not the next day. After our conversation, I decided to get up and try on one of the wigs that my friend Patrice had insisted I purchase in the event that I needed one. I wasn't impressed, so I decided it was not for me. Wearing a wig without hair to fasten it to was uncomfortable. What if while out, it fell off my head? Now this would be rather embarrassing! Deciding that I would stick to my winter trademark of wearing a winter hat with matching scarf, I returned to bed. Revisiting my evening prayers, thanking God for not allowing me to have a pity party, but to truly accept the changes that he had created, I embraced it and accepted this mystery.

Science of the Mind teaches "So you have a problem? This means that you have an opportunity! It means that you have work to do!" Being an early riser, I was up and on my job: reading scriptures, mediating, and planning to meet family and some friends. This helped me to remain focused on the fact that God had already provided for my every need and answered my every prayer. He helped me to better empower myself. This was a way to use this experience as a stepping stone to better things.

About nine AM, my son Regis arrived. He asked, "When are you going to remove your scarf?" With butterflies in my stomach, I slowly removed my scarf. Touching my head, he said, "You look rather cute." Feeling much relief, I thanked him for his words of comfort. We settled down to family business. Later, Mary called and asked if I needed anything? She was on her way. Making a pot of coffee, I awaited her arrival. Asking if I needed anything done in the house, Mary and I settled at our place—the kitchen table. We talked about the "free-floating anxiety" associated with hair loss; we discussed my hair attire versus wearing a wig. Staring at myself in a mirror, with my bald head, really brought it home: Life goes on and I am surviving. We decided to adhere to my original hat-and-scarf plan. We sorted out head gear as we planned my next visit. Good thing it was winter! This headwear would suffice until spring.

When I lifted my vision to God, my outlook became much brighter. By doing this, I was able to be more positive about the remaining chemotherapy sessions. A prayer by St. Richard of Chichester provide me with much hope. It simply states:

Day by Day
Day by day, Dear Lord
Of you,
Three things I pray:
To see you more clearly,
To love you more deeply,
To follow you more nearly,
Day by Day

Now the last leg of the journey had finally arrived. According to the oncologists, the last four treatments would not be as harsh as the first four treatments. The time for each treatment would be longer, but less threatening. For other patients, this might have been true, but not for *moi*. Each treatment was worse than the previous one. The aftermath of each tested my very aching body: joint pains, fever, fatigue, and just plan aching. Each time had me questioning my very existence. Mary accompanied me to each session. Patiently, she sat as I slept, read, ate ice, laughed, and cried. Iva and Clyde kept the driving plan intact. After each therapy, Bea would administer the shot. It is a truism that "Pain is inevitable, but suffering is optional." It was possible that hearing that so often, it had lost some of its meaning. I was just sick of aches and pains. Through spiritual practices, and support of family and friends, I have learned that I was in "the moment," because the worst would be over soon.

At last, the chemotherapy treatments were over. This was a time of celebration. With the accomplishment of each milestone, my friends and family took time to celebrate with me, but this was the *big celebration*. I remembered that one of my friends told me that one day I would look back at this and marvel at my progress and growth; that day was now a reality. At this point, what was walking through my mind was how quickly things can change. Until now, my joys had been few, but today, I felt like a lot had been accomplished. Thanking the staff, Mary and I were given our final instructions. One of which required me to do something special. Maybe it was time to go shopping . I assembled all of my materials. Giving thanks to God for bringing me through the storms and allowing me to climb up the "survival curve" with each portion of treatment I had completed, it was time to go home. There was no doubt that the surgery, reconstruction, and chemotherapy experiences had made an impression on my way of thinking that the quality of my life had indeed changed—for the best.

Change is both the "bane and blessing of life." It brings birth as a reality, as it does death. The good news is that God has blessed me to be counted as a cancer survivor. God gave me a breakthrough. He has sustained me. Psalm 20 says it better: "The Lord answer you in time of trouble. Give victory to the King; Oh Lord, answer us when we call."

I was in a mindset that I had to get through this difficult time to get back to my "normal" life. The oncologist placed me on a prevention medication which will last for five years. God's goodness continually flows into my life, as does healing and success. Breast cancer was not a journey that I had contemplated I would take, but now that I was on the journey, I wanted to understand how to survive the unanticipated circumstances.

Defining this condition or problem has allowed me to experience one of the so-called tests that challenged my faith. Emotionally, I have come to the conclusion that no job is too big for my God. Breast cancer had taken my breast and my hair, but not my spirit or confidence. Family and friends formed my support team. They joke about it now. One thing we all knew was that Satan was a liar. I was not running from the "storms" in my life. I was learning to use the storms to get to a higher place. Reading about other breast cancer survivors, their climbs, and their mountains have helped me during my time of trouble. Breast cancer is a great leveler. I was proud to be in their midst. I have decided to tell my story to warn others to get screenings so they might not have to endure this disease and its treatments.

Continual Decisions

In spite of my *big celebration,* one journey, a new challenge had entered my life. I believed that the grace of God will bring me through whatever circumstances I had to endure, and provide me with all that I ever needed. At all times, his healing would open doors for me. My job was to work to stay alive and do all that I could to ensure that my life was maintained to the best of my ability. I kept my next doctor's appointment. The doctor informed me that I was doing great, and recommended that I consider taking the next step: radiation therapy. You have to understand that this was not on my agenda. Some of the literature I had read did not support the idea of taking this type of treatment. Some said that "radiation increased the risk of secondary cancer in the exposed area." Therefore, I was concerned with the long-term effects of radiation. From the chemotherapy, I was still experiencing nerve damage in my hands and feet. I did not want to create any more long-term discomforts. Since I had completed my chemotherapy, it felt good to have some sense of a "normal" life. I just wanted to be done with treatments of any kind. I was not ready to surrender this freedom. Before leaving the doctor's office, I informed him that I would contact his nurse with my decision. Mary did not say anything. That was a decision that I had to make. This was my journey.

In my thoughts and in my mind, I knew that I was really looking for reasons not to take the next step toward my wellness. It was important to address this issue and not allow it to linger and cause me grief. Going into deep prayers and dialogue with my heavenly father, I prayed for his guidance and wisdom to make the right decision.

*The righteous cry and the Lord heareth and delivered them
out of their troubles.*

(See Psalms 34:17-19.)

As I thought about my decision, in my heart of hearts, I felt that I needed to complete the recommended course of treatment. With this in mind, I decided to call a family conference, so I could get their opinions and reactions. The bottom line decided by their comments was that whatever I decided, they would support me. I talked it over with Mary. We agreed to once again call, make an appointment, and meet with the medical team that would be responsible for this phase of my treatment.

The following week, we set out to keep this appointment, in the lower level of Northwestern Memorial Hospital. This was a far cry from the twenty-first floor, where I had spent the last couple of months taking chemotherapy. Nevertheless, the atmosphere was pleasant and so was the staff. After all the necessary papers were completed, we were introduced to the team members who would be taking care of me. It included the physician, dosimetrist, radiation nurse, and radiation therapist. Then it was necessary to move to the assimilation room. Here the assimilation would demonstrate the radiation procedure. Until I saw this machine, which looked like a body scanner, all was going fine. Since I have an issue with closed-in spaces, I informed the technician that I would not do this exercise. She seemed stunned. Up to this point, we seemed to be getting the procedure completed. Realizing that I was not cooperating, she informed the doctor of the snag. In a few minutes, he returned to the room. After a brief chat and a demonstration of the machine without me in it, he decided to remain in the room until the procedure was completed. This really impressed Mary, the technician, and me. Then the tattoo was explained. Using a black marker, the areas that needed the radiation were marked and secured with surgical tape. This procedure was to ensure that on the day of the treatment, no mistakes would be made.

During the consultation, the doctor explained that a total of thirty-six treatments would be done. Each would last approximately two minutes.

He detailed several side effects that are associated with radiation therapy. According to Dr. Murphy, who defines the side effects as "acute occurring" during treatment or "late occurring" after treatment. They include chronic chest wall pains, dry mouth, and mouth sores that "dramatically affect the day-to-day life." Some research said the quality of life is difficult during the first year of treatment. Armed with all of this information, we completed our consultation. I got dressed. Mary and I headed to breakfast. I thanked everyone for their patience and understanding. We went to the receptionist's desk, scheduled an appointment, and had the parking ticket validated. Our next step was to stop and have a much-needed brunch. We needed to digest Mary's notes. Finally, after driving over to Mary's, I picked up my car and drove home.

Struggling with the issues of treatment, my coping style, and my perception of the treatment had caused some psychological stress. "Knowledge is power" proved to work here. Once I got a better understanding of how this radiation therapy would take place, I felt better. My positive attitude helped me to realize that God would not allow my body to be ravaged by this process. Continuing to pray and meditate on my new set of circumstances, I continued to trust in the Word. Telling myself to "hope in God, for I shall praise him, my help and my God (See Psalms 42:6), I decided to work on a wardrobe for the daily visits to the hospital. I informed my family and children of the pending treatments as my day was coming to an end. The grapevine was busy. In a few minutes, Betty called.

My "traveling angel" was informing me that she wanted to return to be with me during all of my scheduled treatments. "Oh my God!" I screamed into the telephone. I could not believe my ears. He was giving me something that I needed. Giving God praise, I said I know that I can handle this now. Betty stopped my screaming to inform me that she was still on the telephone. As soon as she could check on some reservations, she would get back to me. Being so elated, I reminded her of the saying "God does take care of fools and babies." She just laughed. A few hours later, she called and gave me her itinerary. In the scheme of things, dealing with the condition and not the cause, I could only imagine that having Betty back in this equation would help make things easier on everyone, not just me, but also for Mary, Regis, Sam, and all of the extended family I had come to depend on for so many different things. I thanked Betty for her generosity and caring spirit. We discussed her arrival and who would be there to pick her up. Calm and confident, I prayerfully set my sights on a good night's sleep. It seemed that my journey had just become a little more effortless.

The next morning, as each person called to check on me, I informed each of Betty's decision to return to comfort me in my time of need. Mary and I discussed our travel arrangements. Samantha called and informed me that she would pick Betty up on the date of her arrival. Committed to my *Daily Word, Silent Unity,* other inspirational readings, and meditation, my day was off to a great start. One of the selections stressed the following: "I had been provided with absolutely everything I needed. That God uses all the situations in one's life to get the person where he wants her to go. I thanked him for getting me through the "peaks and valleys." I got busy attempting to spruce up the house for Betty's visit. My other "spiritual vitamins" had provided the energy I needed to become revitalized.

The plans were drawn. For the first week, we would drive to Mary's home. Then Mary would drive us to Northwestern hospital. She wanted to make certain that Betty knew how to get to and from the hospital without getting lost. Then, Mary would take a much-needed and deserved break. For the next thirty days, each morning, Betty would drive me to Northwestern Hospital and wait for me to take treatment. It would take us longer to get there and undress than the treatment lasted. On Mondays, after the treatment, I had to meet with the doctor for his assessment of my progress. Most days, Betty and I stopped for breakfast. Then we would window shop, stop by the library, or just took a walk. Each day, we attempted to do something different. Sometimes, my energy level was high, and other days, I was literally not feeling like engaging in any type of activities. On those days, we did not stay out as long. The treatments were not usually hard. Positioning my arm, during the two minutes, was not comfortable. The technician did attempt to do all that she could to make me comfortable. I worked daily on overcoming any negative tendencies. I decided not to be mentally miserable. Reversing my thinking process helped me to lose the anxiety and fear of the radiation process. Joel Goldsmith wrote, "To be afraid means to empower something or somebody … To not be afraid means you have withdrawn all power from him, her, it, or them." Releasing my fears about radiation therapy by writing about it my journal helped to fight off my anxiety, as much as Betty's presence did.

Of course, the road was not easy, but dealing with the condition and not the cause helped me to face each treatment with more positive energy. Being thankful for Betty's presence, and the support of my friends and family, I shifted my attention to the idea—based on my readings about so many cancer patients before me who had taken radiation treatments and survived—that I would join the list of survivors. The incredible role that Betty played at this stage of my life made me more aware of God's power to surround me with all that I needed to come through this and not to become discouraged. He was the vehicle that had helped me to change my way of thinking.

The radiation treatment was harder for me than the chemotherapy. The texture of my skin as well as the color changed. The doctor said both would return to normal. My vision was affected. As much as I enjoyed reading, my blurry vision would not allow me to enjoy one of the best pastimes of my life. At first, I thought that my eyeglasses needed changing, but did not. The doctor suggested that I wait until I had completed my treatments. My nutritionist suggested that I drink plenty of liquids and eat enough. I offered thanks to Betty and all my caregivers. I was not so wrapped up in my own drama. I thanked God for restoring me and my physical body. Pressing on, my situation became clearer. I realized that I am so blessed because I am surrounded by God's blessings and my healing was taking place. Thank you, Jesus!

"If you have been through what I have been through," as Bishop Paul Morton teaches, you just give God the glory. Realizing that I would be better than ever because God had restored me, I began to experience some of my joy again. That included my hair growing back, my eyesight getting better, and treatments coming to an end. I endured thirty-six treatments, I had not missed one session. I gave God the praise for allowing me to gain my physical and spiritual lessons, placing people, medicine, and medical staff in my life at the right time. He restored me. Despite the frustrations and scary moments, I was still standing.

If things had gone differently, I would not have had the experience of penning the facts of my battle with breast cancer. Being a survivor of breast cancer has helped to prove to my family and friends that there is life after the dismal diagnosis. It also helped to illustrate that having breast cancer did not mean an early coffin. Grounded and spiritually shaped early in life by my parents, Catholic education, family and friends, I have always been committed to a deep interaction and relationship with God, his teachings, and his words. Dealing with breast cancer surgery, reconstruction, chemotherapy, radiation, doctor's visits, aches, pains, physical changes, and the other day-to-day challenges of living has given new meaning to "living the word" in my life.

Eager to get back to new daily routines, I had learned to appreciate just the simple things that I was now able to do. For example, I could bathe myself, go to the beauty salon, my fingernails were growing stronger, and I was driving again. These were things that I had taken for granted. Now, regular visits to the oncologist had gone from monthly to every six months, but Ameridex, cancer medicine, had to be taken for the next five years. Enthused and energized by the success that I was experiencing, I was able to feel good about myself. Help and encouragement from my immediate and extended families, friends, and my concentration on wanting to move forward guided my choices. Recognizing and appreciating the values of growing in faith and the responsibility to continue reaching for a more fulfilled life helped me through those difficult times. My journey might not always have been a direct route, but blessings are often found "on the unexpected detours and rest stops along the way."

Well, one day, while completing my shower, I noticed that my right arm seemed swollen, as well as my fingers. I called the oncologist's office and informed the nurse, Kelly, of my findings. She immediately suggested that I come to the office. Before being discharged from the hospital, part of my briefing included instructions that if I noticed anything strange with the right side of my body, I should call the office. Of course, my next call was to Mary. Informing her of my new encounter. She agreed for us to follow our original script. That is to drive to her home and she would drive to the hospital.

Here we go again. Arriving at the hospital, with mind and spirit intact, it was finally time to see the doctor. Agreeing with my findings, the doctor explained that the swelling indicated that I needed lymphedema treatment. Thanking him for his service, Mary and I departed. The nurse had provided us with a list of out-clinic facilities that provided this sort of treatment. Looking over the list, we located a clinic that was not only closer to my home, but had several openings. I called the facility, and an appointment was made. The therapist called back to suggest that I arrive early so that we could fill out the necessary papers and have the measurements taken before the therapy session. Driving myself to the clinic, I said, "Thank you, God, for my blessings!" Only his goodness had allowed me to find new hope and courage in what seemed to be a new discomfiting experience. As usual, I had an early-morning appointment. Arriving at the site, I completed all of the necessary forms. Then my name was called and I was introduced to my therapist.

She explained to me the details of the therapy sessions, and concluded by doing the first of my eight scheduled treatments. The treatment included physical therapies, massages, apply lotion, and wrapping. The wrapping was to remain for at least twenty-four hours or as long as I could keep it on. This turned out to be the worst part. At each visit, measurements would be taken to determined if the swelling was going away. At first it was terribly hard to keep the bandage on all night. After about fifteen hours, it had to come off. Then finally I could get some sleep. This process went for eight treatments. At the end of the eighth treatment, I would be measured for a fitted sleeve that when worn would help to minimize the swelling. Knowing that God was my safety net, I released any thoughts of this discomfort and allowed the healing process to take over.

Experiencing more opportunities to say "yes" to life and continuing on my road to mending, I scheduled a trip to Louisiana and Texas. I had promised Betty whenever I was able to travel, she would be the first one I visited. Emotionally, I had gone from "rags to riches." My success was not defined by my own accomplishments, but by God's loving grace. Proceeding with resolve and profound faith in the Spirit of the journey, the distance at times seemed long, but as the young people say, "it's all good."

According to research and other cancer survivors, cancer can be an isolating experience. Helping to make my experience bearable were my friends, immediate and extended families. Once my secret was out, and some people stopped being angry, I had extra support. They sustained me through treatments and beyond. Slowly, as my body issues and other issues began to subside, I was ready to focus on living again. Gradually, I stopped waiting for the other proverbial shoe to drop. I stopped feeling like a cancer victim and started behaving like a cancer survivor.

Broadly defined, a cancer survivor is anyone who has been diagnosed with any type of cancer. Last fall, the Institute of Medicine detailed shortfalls in survivors' cases. In its key recommendations, the institute proposed that every cancer patient receive a "survivorship care plan." Such a plan, for adult survivors of childhood cancers, already is in place. It is called STAR (Survivors Taking Action and Responsibility). At least once a year, patients are seen to monitor effects of past treatments, and when necessary, referred to specialist. Northwestern Memorial Hospital is considering a similar clinic for survivors of adult cancer.

As with so many Americans who have survived breast cancer, I continue to experience nerve damage in my hands and feet. I am less sensitive to heat or cold, but more vulnerable to frostbite. After treatment, I thought that all of my limbs would be restored to some sort of normalcy, but this did not happen. So far, I do not have what some people call "chemo brain." That is when women survivors of breast cancer suffer from deficits in memory, concentration, and executive functioning. While weight loss is a common side effect of cancer during treatment, I was not so favored. Sometimes I wished that I was. Why? Oh, I had this vision of a complete wardrobe makeover, which included smaller sizes and jazzier clothing. Believe me, it was just a dream. I did not lose one pound. Instead, during one phase of the chemotherapy, I gained a couple of extra pounds. According to the doctor, that was medicine-related. Chemotherapy and the steroid medication were responsible for this weight increase. As soon as this medicine was no longer needed, the weight disappeared. Thanks to better eating habits, more walking, and learning to take better care of myself, I did avoid a lot of additional weight.

Trusting "Divine Order," I have affirmed that healing is working throughout my body. I have learned whenever I am having anxious moments to turn my thoughts to God and ask for his intercession. Realizing that from the depth of my being, my experiences were processes that I had to undergo to deepen my connection with God and heighten my awareness of God within me. I focused on his presence, learned to relax, opened my mind, and dismissed some of my concerns, which allowed me the time I needed to listen for inspirations from God and the answers to my prayers. Now, as I look back on what seemed like an impossible time in my life, the stress, the frustration and exhaustion, all were necessary actions to make necessary changes. During this time, I have learned a lot. To begin, making self-care my top priority and to develop a more personalized spiritual practice kept me focused on my faith and healing.

The Next Dimension

The spiritual states "what I cannot do for myself, Jesus will do for me because he loves me. is very encompassing." Using my "weapons of mass destruction," including but not limited to faith in the word of God, caring, nurturing, family, friends, and all of my prayer partners have given me insight into my spiritual growth. I am bouncing back with a fierce determination and motivated to share with everyone how blessed I really am, empowered to be totally at peace with the new me. Rev. Dr. Floyd Flakes simply puts it like this: "because God loves me, I can have a victory celebration."

How easy it is to forget that we are involved in spiritual warfare (Eph. 6:12). We cannot blame Satan for everything, but we should be aware of his influence. Quietly talking with my Father in heaven, giving thanks rather than complaining, I know that he understands my hurts and will graciously bring healing to my body. In one of Dottie Peoples's songs of inspiration, she sings "forever grateful for your grace and your mercy... if it wasn't for Your grace and mercy... thank you for your grace and mercy." My old life was over and a time of intense transformation had begun.

During one of my many readings, I read that a belief is something you hold, but a conviction is something that holds you. Assumptions are the foundation stones. Principles are the actual building blocks. This helped me to understand that I was building on what God has equipped me with to function effectively according to my spiritual gifts. God knew that I need a power greater than myself to withstand Satan, so he has provided himself living in me. "Greater is he who is in you than he who is in the world" (see John 4:4). Fred Hammond said it better: "God did it."

Trusting in the statement, "wherever I am, God is, and all is well," I reaffirmed that my faith would make all things possible.

Some may read this and think that I am living in a fantasy world or a world of make-believe. No, I am not. Yes, people are still dying from cancer, and research has not found a cure, but the possibilities are endless. If I continue to have faith and practice what I believe "... all things shall be added unto you." (See Matt. 6:33.) Not flaunting my spiritual beliefs but living them has established an atmosphere that has bolstered my faith. Silent Unity teaches that as "our meditation and prayers work deeper, we begin to have moments where we feel in the flow of life." This affirmation: *Believe that you have already received it, and it will be yours* summed up how my network of personal friends extended across the nation, families, and Silent Unity prayer partners helped to strengthen and gain greater control over this new life experience.

Praying, trusting God, and doing my best, I thanked him for his mercy. Thank you, Jesus, because I know it is you and not me. "For by graces are ye saved; it is the gift of God... for we are his workmanship, which God hath before ordained that we should walk in them (Eph. 2:8-10). In faith, I prayed that God's unending blessing would make me well, both physically and emotionally. Trusting in God, I see myself as a child of his who is showered with unlimited blessings that I have gained through greater spiritual understanding and a renewed awareness of mind, body, and soul. God continues to hold me in his hands.

Having family and friends pray and comfort me has made it possible for me to make it through treatments, fears, and anxiety. With God's approval, I was determined not to allow doubt or fear to take away my blessings.

My story is still being written. I thank God every day that he has allowed me to recognize the fear and doubt, but to get through them. There is no question that "from my lips to God's ears," praying to complete treatments and just day-to-day survival as a breast cancer survivor was made easier by the love and compassion of my friend, Mary, cousin Betty, Regis, daughter-in-law, Samantha, family members, and a host of friends.

"Call it a clan,
call it a network,
call it a tribe,
call it a family.
Whatever you call it,
Whoever you are,
You need one."
Jean Howard, *Families*

With so many decisions and choices to make, it was much easier for me because family and friends were there to help me to make the best decisions for myself

Life's trials and tragedies happened for a reason. In fact, God gives us "tools" to learn the lessons that are needed. A spiritual teacher, Eckhart Tolle offers to all the faithful this simple message of hope. "There is a way out of suffering and into peace." Taking time each day to turn to God in prayer has helped me to develop a more peaceful spirit and sense of direction. Loren Cummingham and David Hamilton's *Why Not Women?* said that "God won't crush you. He will give you enough grace to fulfill what he has called you to do." *The Science of Mind* teaches that "the Spirit can only give us what we can take." And since praying is a mental process, it is necessary for us to accept that the Spirit has already provided everything.

God has been gracious. Having breast cancer has presented an opportunity for me to "sweep out the old and make room for the new." Having breast cancer has helped to make me more appreciative of what life has to offer. Learning to cope with the problems or trials associated with being a breast cancer survivor have aided in my "new blueprint" for a better way of living. Learning to reduce stress, adopting healthier nutritional habits, and exercising more have helped me to develop a better way of life. With commitment, awareness, meditation, and spiritual empowerment, I have adopted affirmations and strategies that helped to alleviate my pains and worries. Dr. Jeremiah Wright, Sr., pastor of Trinity Unity Church of Christ, puts it this way: "When the tears flowed, it opened up the channels where healing needs to take place, which is a sign of being strong and dealing with life's problems. In the midst of instability, God is still in charge; morning by morning.

All that I have needed, God has provided. God has brought me to the end of a season and opened a new season.

Having CT and bone scans produced no metastasis to my bones, lungs, or liver, which are the first three places cancer usually spreads. That gave me a lot to be thankful for. My chemo "cocktails"—eight intravenous doses or the "red devil" as dubbed by others for its resemblance to cherry Kool-Aid—coupled with all its nasty side effects helped me to give thanks to God who has blessed my life abundantly. Many breast cancer veterans advised diets similar to that of pregnant women; eat many small meals, extra proteins, limited fatty and oily foods, lots of ginger and peppermint. I have learned to take their advice and developed healthier eating habits. Learning to better appreciate the day-to-day experiences of my life, I now have a more enjoyable life. Spiritual teacher Eckhart Tolle offers all in faith a simple message of hope: "There is a way out of suffering and into peace."

There were times on this journey of coping and surviving that I looked at the world and my surroundings with envy and regret. Imagining that everyone else had been given a more fulfilling and enjoyable life was not good for me. At times, I was very uncomfortable with myself and my surroundings. One thing that I did learn is that "worrying is a misuse of the imagination." Therefore, I had to reach deep down into my bag of spiritual belief and take the problem to God in prayer. I know that I have a good friend in Jesus. I relied on God's words, in Matthew 28:20, "surely I am with you always to the end of ages." Faith, love, blessing and an incredible medical team have allowed me to reach this phase of my life. Accepting the fact that the Spirit has already provided me with everything that I need, I rely on the word of God to guide me. Releasing all into the name of Jesus, I know who knows what to do. Jesus is the way, the truth, and the light.

Spiritual Reflections

Thriving on the words of God, I had a radical transformation. With an eye on the cycles of life, a time for growth, and a time for death, with stops in between, I have developed new ideas and inspirations to energize me daily. Anything is possible with God. Whatever he wants me to do, "his will be done." Moving forward, I had to find a way to fight. Though sometimes I wished for an opportunity to return to "the good old days," these are now my "good old days." It was normal to be afraid, but working to keep abreast of the new research information, treatment choices, and maintaining my regular doctor appointments, I have a chance to support my wellness—mind, body, and spirit. There is a spiritual song that says "what I cannot do for myself, Jesus will do for me because he loves me." God is getting me ready for a new season in my life.

Returning to some of my volunteering with Catholic Charities, VASA (Volunteer for Senior Advocacy) and serving as president of the Chicago Bronzeville Lions Club have helped me to accept my challenges and live as normal a life as possible. In addition to these endeavors, I am the proud grandmother of Lisette, the newest addition to my family. Leaning on another of the affirmations of *Silent Unity* "as our meditation and prayer deepen, we begin to have moments where we feel in the flow of life." My daily survival became much more tolerable. In addition, Yvette Gunn's *The Blessings Behind Tribulations* gives a list of things to work on while God works through your crisis to bearing you victory. "... `a victory so big, you will look back one day and not remember your crisis, except to share your testimony of how the Lord delivered you!"

WHAT TO DO WHILE YOU ARE GOING THROUGH THE FIRE:

1. When something major happens, talk to God first;
2. Don't tell everyone what you're experiencing;
3. Talk to a trustworthy friend who is knowledgeable in the Word and vent to that person only;
4. Confess the Word of God over your situation. The more you speak God's word over your situation, the more God can work in your life.

BY FOLLOWING THESE SEVEN STEPS, YOU WILL SEE THESE BLESSINGS MANIFEST IN YOUR LIFE.

1. God will draw closer to you because your trust and honor him first;
2. Your love for God will increase;
3. Your faith will increase;
4. You will get better at hearing God's voice and heeding his guidance.
5. Your examples will be an encouragement to others;
6. You will have a beautiful testimony to tell when the Lord delivers you out of the situation;
7. Your testimony will give God the glory.

It might sound crazy at times, but by faith, it has to work. Remember, God promises us that he will never leave us or forsake us. (See Hebrews 13:5.) Whenever you have that embedded in your heart, you can move forward with confidence. Speaking God's words over my circumstances helped me to see the manifestation of him working in my life. And this was taking place before my introduction to Yvette Gunn's writing.

When experiencing a major crisis, one of the most important factors to remember is that it is temporary. As 2 Corinthians 5:18 states, "while we look not at the things which are seen but at things which are not seen. For the things seen are temporal, but the things which are not seen are eternal." There were some things that I thought would hold me down, but once I gave them to God in prayer, my vision became clearer. Holding on to God's unchanging hand and word, I came to understand who I am in the Word of Jesus. This I know, God will supply my every need.

A philosopher once wrote that he could not believe in a God who did not know how to dance. Reading this, I laughed aloud. The more I thought about it, I could follow the philosopher's thought pattern, because as in dancing, a part of prayer is learning how to listen, so as to feel the rhythm. It is also paying attention to what is going on, both inside and outside. Learning to lean on God to direct my steps was a way of connecting and interacting with him. God leading and my following could be contrasted with dancing. God guides and leads me. He moves in strategic ways and with a purpose in my life. (See Psalm 23). He never guides or leads where there is not a goal, growth or outcome.

Thriving on the Word of God, I had a fresh perspective on my journey and was energized for the long haul. It is easy to place too much time into feeling discouraged. Putting my faith and trust in God meant that some things take time; not my time, but his time. It will all work out in the end! Perseverance and patience are results of seeing the big picture; God is in charge. Learning to use the weapons that God has given to set me free or not miss out on what he has planned for me, as in Romans 5:3-4, the apostle Paul said, "… let us exalt him and triumph over our troubles and rejoice in our suffering, knowing that pressure and affliction and hardship produce patient and un answering endurance…"

Dr. Bridgett Hilliard says, "If you can understand faith and learn to live by the word, you can overcome any challenge in life that you are faced with." This parallels the teaching in another one of her books, *My Thoughts on Victorious Confession.* She expounds, "Learn how to take God's Word, apply it to your life and speak it out of your mouth and stop speaking all of the negative things out of your mouth." I would love it if I could put it in a pill and get people to learn to live by faith. This is the whole essence of life; learning to live by faith and live by what the Word of God says. The Bible tells us that at one time we were all dead in sin and blind to the truth of God. As the hymn "Amazing Grace" states, "I once … was blind but now I see." In Ephesians 1:18, it states, "he healed the eyes of our hearts so that we can see. So thanking

God for his healing touch has helped me to tell others about his healing power in my life. God's spiritual promises have comforted me and given me hope. Trusting "Divine Order," I have affirmed that healing was working throughout my body. I have learned whenever I am having anxious moments to turn my thoughts to God and ask for his blessings and comfort.

Bishop T. D. Jakes "80/20" rule painted a picture that sticks with me. He simply said it this way. "Nothing is going to give you 100 percent of anything in life." At times, 80 percent might look smaller than 20 percent because the focus is on the 20 percent that you do not have. Informing God about the 20 percent that you do not have takes more away from the 80 percent that you have been granted. Think about it! Bishop Jakes recommended spending time on the 80 percent that you have, and the 20 percent that is missing won't seem so important. This battle with breast cancer has given me a chance to completely revitalize and better my spirituality. This might sound corny and maybe too philosophical or something to that effect, but that is how I view my spiritual being. This has allowed me to break free from some ways of thinking that were not blessing me and making my life difficult. But God never promised an easy life; he promised a blessed life.

Rev. Tony preached a sermon that said when you position yourself with God, he will invade your situation and bring a solution. "The Lord will fulfill his purpose for me; thy steadfast love. Oh Lord, endures forever. Do not forsake the work of thy hands." (See Psalm 138) Suffering is a stepping stone to a loving relationship with God. This I read and believe; therefore, I turned to the "author of my life" (See Acts 3:15) to take me to the next level. How good God is!

In such time of stress or personal illness, praying remains a powerful weapon. Remembering what God has done stabilized me and placed my feet on solid ground. Looking to the Blessed Mother's intercession, I began to pray to Our Lady of Lourdes Special Mass for Healing. The Miracles of Lourdes began in 1858, at a grotto near a little village in Southwestern France. Mary appeared to a young woman named Bernadette eighteen times, announcing "I am the Immaculate Conception." Mary helped Bernadette to discover a hidden spring at the grotto. That spring was soon to become a fountain of faith, hope, and healing for millions of pilgrims who visit there each year.

Lourdes is truly a place of healing. The Catholic Church recognizes sixty-five miraculous cures there, and thousands more have been reported. My brother enrolled me in the Lourdes Prayer League masses that are held monthly at the Shrine of Our Lady of Lourdes in France, and each day at the National Shrine of Our Lady of the Snows in Belleville, Illinois. Another novena prayer that my family and friends have said daily is the Precious Blood Novena Prayer. The purpose of this novena prayer was "to beseech God to help us whom he has redeemed with his Precious Blood."(New revised *Jesus, Mary and Joseph Manual*). A Novena for Peace of Mind, by the Sacred Heart League, said daily asking God to find peace and acceptance in the midst of difficult situations because trust in his word provided me peace in my thoughts, words, and actions. The Prayers to St. Jude, which is a prayer for the intercession of St. Jude for serious problems when feeling hopeless and alone, and for desperate cases, have been a part of life and used more each day as I make the best of times out of the worst of times. "It is the Lord who gives wisdom; out of his mouth comes knowledge and understanding." (See Proverbs 2:6.)

Words of praise, inspirations, and meditations have illustrated that prayers have always united me to God. Finally, realizing that I have drawn closer to God just by redefining my spiritually and praying for wisdom to make the best of life now and faith in life to come. Praying for guidance, understanding, and insight, I follow "all the Scripture." (See Luke 24:27.) Not wanting to abuse the precious gift of life that I had been given, I thank God for being in the midst and reminding me that I had learned a valuable lesson for my situation; that I am protected through all situations. Joyce Meyer teaches that when you pray, you open the door for God to work in your life. John 11:40 states only believe and you will see... Every day, God's working on my behalf, and I shall see the results. I am going to trust God to help me, because I know he is my answer.

Challenges of Coping

Helen Keller once wrote, "Be of good cheer. Do not think of today's failures, but of the success that may come tomorrow. You have yourself a difficult task, but you will succeed if you persevere; and you will find joy in overcoming obstacles. Remember no effort that we make to attain something beautiful is ever lost." These are powerful words from a woman who definitely knew struggle.

Breast cancer has a far-reaching and permanent effect on survivors. There has to be a clear understanding and knowledge of breast cancer and all of its facets. Dr. Sandra Million Underwood, RN, PHD, FAAAN, a well-known breast cancer specialist and activist, says, "Understand the science behind the disease and treatment. Today's medicine is entirely different and more advanced than in the past. All of the medications that we are utilizing now are the results of clinical trials." Breast cancer is an emotionally challenging disease. There are so many options and choices that are left to the individual.

New treatments and scientific studies are released on a regular basis. Years ago, doctors treated all breast cancer procedures the same way: perform a mastectomy and that was it. Now doctors tailor treatments to the individual patient. When healthy diets and lifestyles are present, the desired healing's chances are much better. Depending on the amount of surgery, follow-up procedures, and treatments, breast cancer survivors' survival skills are very important. Understanding the challenges and how to overcome them is dealing with reality. Healthy survivorship has a clear definition. Wendy Harpham, author of *Diagnosis Cancer*, says "a survivor who gets good care and lives as fully as possible is a healthy survivor." She adds, "Finding a balance between hope and acceptance;

preparing for likely outcome while hoping for the best; in other words choosing life and living until you die and not a day sooner."

While it may sound simplistic, it is not. Cancer forces its survivors to make choices they might not want to make, under conditions that are not pleasant. Remembering that I had read, "no one can handle such an experience as breast cancer and not get angry is a mistake," has aided in my survival. Counting my blessings, successful surgery, great medical support, family and friends who gave 100 percent of themselves; walking and doing for myself, I praise God for his mercy and favor. Sometimes I think that having breast cancer has caused me more stress than the two recognized common causes of recorded stress. They are listed as career changes and moving. These experiences I felt that I had some control over, but breast cancer was quite different. This is one stress that I did not control. But God, who supplies my every need or want, and who has brought me this far, provided the words that I needed to address my situation. As I became less frustrated, I noticed that my coping skills were improving. Learning to celebrate each stage helped me to let go and move forward. Watching the birds soar or the flower buds unfold, I could not give up. Something in me made me want to live and not give up. Bishop Paul Morton's "You Restored Me," "On High Alert," and "Making Something Look Like It's Not" are just three spiritual inspiration songs that inspired me to feel stronger and in control.

A feeling of debilitating tiredness or total lack of energy that lasts for days, weeks, or even longer is the most common side effect of chemotherapy. More than nausea, pain, or depression, the mental and physical discomforts of treatments can be worst. Cancer fatigue is real and it's different than what healthy people feel at the end of a long day. And unlike usual tiredness, post-cancer fatigue is not released with a good night's rest, but rather it is a chronic challenge of "balancing work and life to function."

Learning to listen to my body, exercise, nutrition, spiritual activities, and not pushing my limits have been very much a part of my daily survival strategy. Also, part of the good news is that I have not had to learn coping skills on my own. Learning to cope was a gift of God's goodness and mercy. Like the Psalmist, my heart sang with thanksgiving. "You changed my mourning into dancing; you took off my sackcloth and clothed me with gladness. With my whole being, I sing endless praise to you. Oh Lord my God, forever will I give thanks" (Psalms 30:12-13).

Knowing that he supports me in all my trials and endeavors, learning to cope as well as deal with the barriers have made for a better life.

According to a very popular and familiar passage of scripture, "for everything there is a time and season for every matter under the sun." The countless obstacles, aches, pains, and other side effects of dealing with breast cancer have been more acceptable because of the love, prayers, and nurturing that I have experienced with God, who set me up to get up and move on. There are many avenues that I could have taken, but turning to God in prayer was the simplest and easiest thing for me. Included in my litany of prayers are those to Saint Michael of the Saints Trinitarian Mystic & Cancer Patrons, Prayers for Cancer patients and Prayers to the Mother of Sorrow Through the Intercession of Saint Peregrine, patron of cancer victims. Praying helped me to feel more connected to God, who is my "constant source of healing." The choice was simple. Either I would become hardened against God "who has allowed this to happen to me," or I would become "softened and ultimately release my concerns to him." I affirm: "God *is my light and where there is light there can be no darkness.*" With perseverance, dedication, and desire to succeed, I continued praying for God to give me strength to cope with being a cancer survivor with chronic illness. I agree with Lynn Redgrave: "Being a cancer survivor is the most challenging role of my life."

"Many are the plans in a man's heart, but it is the Lord's purpose that prevails." (See Proverb 19.) Some adults have a saying that life is not easy. They continue to say that it is filled with difficulties, strife, and problems. Senior citizens are faced with another set of challenges. This is the group that I now identify with at this time in my life. All of the problems that are associated with becoming a senior citizen, I have encountered: fixed income, graying hair, arthritic pains. But having breast cancer was not one that I envisioned. Here are a few updated facts about breast cancer.

According to the American Cancer Association, some breast cancer facts are:

- Nearly 80 percent of breast cancer is found in women over fifty.
- Risk factors include family history; previous abnormal biopsy; first period before age twelve or menopause after fifty-five; having no children or first child after age thirty; heavy alcohol use; and obesity.
- The U.S. has more than 2 million breast cancer survivors.
- In the U.S., breast cancer is the most common diagnosed cancer among African-American women.
- There is a new diagnosis every three minutes, and a life lost every fourteen minutes.
- At age 40, Caucasian women are more likely to be diagnosed with breast cancer than African American women.
- Up to 10 percent of breast cancer is believed to be inherited.

Jesus said worry prohibits spiritual growth. (See Luke 8:14.) Therefore, it is important to understand how to deal with common worries. Some of life's circumstances are beyond my control, like breast cancer. But what I have learned to do was to place the situation in God's hands. That included prayerful planning, family and friends praying for a positive outcome and prayer groups praying for my well-being. Studies have indicated that 30 percent of worries are beyond our abilities to change. The Scriptures give four very important reasons why worries should be taken to God in prayer:

(1) Because God already knows my needs and worries (See Matt. 6, 8, 31);
(2) Because God is able to meet my needs and remove my worries (See Matt. 6:26,28-30); (3) Because God wants

to provide for me (See 1 Pet. 5:7); and (4) Because prayer produces results (See Phil. 3: 6-7).

The daunting task of facing the aftermath of breast cancer is reaffirming that my faith would help me to learn to cope. By expanding my consciousness to a wider vision, out of this uncertain period in my life revealed a clearer direction that would help to move me forward. "Pray that according to the riches of his glory, he may grant that you may be strengthened in your inner being." (See Ephesians. 3:16) During this time of personal challenge, with breast cancer, I have learned to center my thoughts in a spirit of thankfulness on just two words: "God is." Mary L. Kudpferle says, "God works through many channels to heal. God is your health. God is your strength. God is your guidance. God is your peace.

Whatever you need, God is the fulfillment of that need here and now and always! Remember and be assured:

> The light of God surrounds you;
> The love of God enfolds you;
> The power of God watches over you;
> Wherever you are, God is."

With a renewed sense, each day I want my life to be full and complete; therefore, I had to learn to let go of old worries and accept the now. Another of my favorite songs, "The Lord Is Blessing Me Right Now," infuses me with hope and faith. Reading in one article that the Lord has no desire to make me miserable physically, emotionally, or spiritually and learning to experience genuine spiritual growth, have improved my decision and attitude to consider what is best for my survival. My personal conviction is that God answers prayers, and I am living proof. A poem by James Dillet Freeman, "Oneness" helped to instill in me that God is in charge. It made me realize more than ever that I am God's creation. Simply it states "…I am the cup and You are poured in me, through me, over me Lord."

Gaining a better understanding of the effects of breast cancer and learning what is necessary to fight this battle have been great discoveries for me. Still working with God and giving him my problems has allowed me to rely on his words to be my guide. He said, with you until the end of the ages. (See Matthew 28:20) Several affirmations that have helped me to cope are :

"I face each day with a smile and the day smiles at me."

"Faith keeps me strong and calm in the storm of life."

"Let go, Let God."

"God's will. God's way."

"Thank God for the blessings of a perfectly functioning body."

"Trusting in God, I am blessed throughout my journey of life."

"For you need endurance, so that when you have done the will of God, you may receive what he has promised." (See Hebrews 10:36) Guiding through slippery situations in life can be a challenge. I affirm that God is the stabilizing force in my life that enables me to remain steady and serene. Working flawlessly in my life, I feel the results of greater peace and God's love. Experiencing life at the deepest level of self-reflection converted my fears into faith and empowered my spiritual growth.

Depending on who you talk with, much has been written about survival rates, and there is no discussion about quality-of-life issues when it is assumed that mastectomy leads to the poorest quality of life. Selecting the mastectomy with reconstruction and five years of the little white pill, I have had a wonderful outcome and have never regretted my decisions. Still I believe more can be done to help survivors once their treatments are over. Teaching cancer survivors using the "whole patient" approach is important for the survivor to get the most appropriate and effective treatments needed, because cancer drugs often have side effects. Understanding the impact of cancer on the body, mind, and all that it entails, learning to cope is a challenge.

Follow-up visits sometimes pulled me where my spirit did not want to go. Sometimes I had to revisit those emotions which caused fear, anxiety, and made me jumpy.

Who would not be nervous? Sliding past the number-two killer illness is no laughing matter. Learning over time that worrying about a relapse or recurrence of cancer makes little or no difference in my health. It does not help the quality of my life. Psychologists tell us that worrying in and of itself has no benefit if it is not translated into positive action. Brian Stables, Ph.D. recommends that you listen to your body.

Put yourself on a worry diet. Day by day, cut down on amount of time you let yourself have to worry. He claims that this does work.

As more and more survivors live longer and indeed recover from breast cancer, healthcare teams will have to address the aftermath of breast cancer and its treatments. Talking with a professional about breast cancer and its impact on life often helps healing. Accurate information about the disease and its treatment aids recovery. Talking to women who have completed breast cancer therapy provides encouragement and insight into treatment, in a way that your healthcare team cannot always do. Keeping active and listening to your body's needs are tools for coping with breast cancer.

But as the number of survivors has soared to more than 10 million, many have become activists, demanding not just first-rate medical care but also recognition and management of the physical, emotional, and fallouts from breast cancer and its treatment. Still today, the best method of coping despite the many contradictory scientific releases about breast cancer, is to pray and move on. This way, I am able to learn more about the disease, and not give up. I pray that one day "we'll say breast cancer is a chronic disease, a thing that you don't die from but can live with." These are the words of Soraya, a spirited songwriter who lost her breasts to cancer. Many problems you can think of did not come to stay. They came to pass away, in the name of Jesus. Sickness did not come to stay in your life. Jesus declared, "Heaven and earth shall pass away, but my words shall not pass away." (See Matt. 24:35.) The Word of God is going to dominate this area of my life. "... And his Word will *never, never pass away!*"

When learning to cope with the challenges, here are some of the things that I have learned from my own experiences and that of others, as well as from the advice of professionals. First, this is serious. Treat it as such. Do not try to go on as if nothing has happened to you. Educate yourself. Start searching for information on how to manage the illness; how others coped.

Deeper Dimensions

A philosopher once wrote that he could not believe in a God who didn't know how to dance. The change of season, traditions, and experiences are in constant motion. The changes , growth and outcome of all things that are prayed for are because of God's power. Acknowledging God in my life, I know he moves in strategic ways. This said to me that nothing just happens. Whatever happens was with purpose (Psalm 23). He guides me and leads me. He is guiding me. He never guides us where there is no goal He never asks me to get up from where I am unless he shows me how to do it. The constant interaction of God in my life through prayer is little like dancing. God leads and I follow.

As in dancing, a part of prayer is learning how to listen, learning to feel the rhythm. It's paying attention to what's going on both inside and outside, and letting God direct how it goes, and guide. Someone once said that endings never end before new beginnings start. The fact that old circumstances are moving out should be accepted as a sign that new and better circumstances are on the way. Counting on the Spirit to handle my situations, I know that God does not have to explain what he does or how he does it. Whatever comes in my life is part of God's master plan. He allows all of the disruptions to come because what he has in store is much greater than what was before the season of change. Leaning on what I know has been around for years, God, who "upholds and sustains me," it is the life of God within that allowed me to focus on the positive outcome, rather than negative circumstances. God is to me just what I will let him be: my strength and my rock.

"Things we have to go through," Rev. Dr. Frank E. Ray preaches that being a chosen, a child of God, the God we serve walks with me, talks with me, "not as either or..." God knows all about our sickness, needs, and wants. God wants to get the best out of us. He carries us through some things, one step at a time. I feel, first of all, very, very, very blessed that I feel rather healthy. Realizing as difficult as things have been, I am just grateful to be given the privilege of experiencing all that I have been exposed to and receive in gratitude. During one of her telecasts, Joyce Meyer pointed out that "with God, all things are possible. His strength is made perfect in our weakness. God is a miracle-working God."

One cancer survivor suggested, "Focus on the important ones and decide what you can handle. One thing is planning and sticking to the top three items on the list and letting everything else go." Keeping the goal of flexibility in mind and asking God to give me strength, peace, and courage, my life seemed to be coming together. Out of stress and fear came guidance. Challenges, problems, and crises are a part of everyday life, but more so when you are a cancer survivor. For some, a breast cancer survivor gaining confidence in the ability to overcome personal issues and re-establishing an everyday life pattern can be very hard.

Even in the confusion of life, God knows what he is doing. Reading a journal that said cancer falls most heavily on the elderly, which is a rising population in the United States, really hit home. Another report discussed that cancer "is rarely a solo act." It said that cancer doesn't exist in a vacuum. At least half the people who are diagnosed with cancer already suffer from other illness, or co-morbidity, such as heart disease, diabetes, hypertension, or arthritis, some of which could be life-threatening in their own right. One researcher reported that specific conditions directly impacted whether a woman was diagnosed with breast cancer earlier or later in life. Overall, investigators found that mammography screening and contact with the medical care system decreased the probability of late-stage diagnosis.

After reading all of the above information, I thought if I had known all of this before, I would have inquired earlier about my chances of having breast cancer. No sense in saying what could have been; the fact is, I am blessed and will take better care of myself. One thing I am sure of is that I am not alone. Praying this prayer, "God I know you are in charge of my life," during one of my morning meditations have helped to anchor my thoughts and reactions. Does this sound like a bold statement to you? It once did to me, but let me assure you, there is a peace that comes over me when I allowed the guidance of God to take me to the next step. Learning how to "rise above the waters, the heavy sea cannot threaten us nor can the mighty water upset us, for we are free from fear." Letting go and letting God assures that the "peace of God, which surpasses understanding" is a gift and a part of God's lavish and abundant love. (See Phil. 4:7.)

Sometimes, prayers were a "tranquilizer," something taken only when faced with challenging circumstances or in unfamiliar territory. Some people lose their faith, and others find it. Asking God to help me understand what he was doing in my life, all I know was I believed him.

Prayer is not a "pill" to take. Prayer is an act of thought and feeling, in which you allow what is in you to express itself through you to out there, as explained by Charles Roth. He said that when an emergency or unexpected threatening circumstances suddenly came into your life, the first thing to do is to turn your mind in the direction of God's presence and power. Bernice Ketchum said, "Practice praying just as you would music." This exercise only takes five minutes and it can be done anywhere. Procrastination! Make a decision not to rain on your own parade. Take the steps necessary to begin with a slate clean of whatever, whether it is a simple decision, a phone call to make, or a conversation you need to have to get the ball rolling.

That prayer can have health benefits now appears sufficiently well-supported by research data that the American Cancer Society recently declared. "Sometimes answers come from prayers when medical science has none." Some physicians and academics protested when the American Cancer Society made that statement. But the Cancer Society's statement was influenced by the increasing body of research that suggests that when you pray for yourself, you are doing something medically wise. Martin Seligman, former president of the American Psychological Association, has supposed that prayer helps recovery from illness and depression by focusing the mind on things to be grateful for in life.

Knowing that God is the unlimited resources from which all goodness comes, affirms that turning to God in times of fear or anxiety is beneficial to me. Understanding that challenges or even problems are a part of life, that is the work of God. That work of God is to "wake me up so that one can learn to hear what God is saying and prepare to do his Work." Finally, reading and learning that prayer itself is the work of God, I planned and allowed moments of prayer daily, which nurtures me and makes for a better day.

What I like about prayer is that there is no set formula for calling on God. I am free to send any message that I want! I can just say hello or just "thanks" for all the things he has done for me. On the other hand, I can express how things are going astray and I need reinforcement. Having a relationship with God, through prayers, has been my constant relief of all my discouragements and baffling breast cancer experiences.

Never underestimating the power of prayer, because of the power of prayer, my life was changed. Also, it parted the Red Sea. It raised the dead. It has always brought victory wherever it has gone. That's what prayer has done and will continue to do. James 5:16 says, "The effectual fervent prayer of a righteous man availeth much." There is power in prayer that is available to everyone. The Word of God is a "suit of armor more solid and sturdy than any of those that you have ever seen with your physical eye."

Prayer is an act of thought and feelings in which I allow what is in me to express itself through me to the "out there." It is a special kind of mind activity or thinking. It is a thinking that is directly pointed toward God; to a power which is a "transcendent presence and a power to which you are connected."

The Honorable Minister Louis Farrakhan says that "pain is the mother of change." All of us go through things in life when we ask the question, "why?" God said in the Bible that "my ways are not your ways. My thoughts are not your thoughts." God wants me to come out victorious even in my time of change with breast cancer. The devil might have a plan for my defeat, but God always has a plan for my victory. He wants to restore me. God has no other job to do, purpose, or responsibility than to lead an outcome that is best for me.

Intellectually, *Science of the Mind* continues to nourish me with the wisdom of its founder Ernest Holmes and its teaching. Learning to apply the philosophy in my everyday life, through meditation and spiritual practices, I am still climbing and reaching my goals. God has taught me to understand that whatever I am going through, I am blessed. God made me tough long before things got rough. He made me to want ease and happiness, but God taught me how to stand when no one else was standing. He taught me how to take care of myself. He was getting me ready to sing my song. He taught me how to sing solo a long time ago. He made a way for me. I will survive. He made me tough. He groomed me with a daddy who told me that I was somebody. What God had planned for my life helped me to choose his way and him in my life. If it had not been for him, I would have lost my mind. I would not have made it this far. My soul cries Alleluia. I bless his holy name. With the Lord on my side, he keeps on making a way for me. Thank you, God, for how you take care of me. He keeps on blessing me. Each day has brought its own blessings into my life. I could have been wiped out, but for some reason he saw fit to keep me here to give this testimony.

Moving Forward

In this book, I have shared and explored breast cancer, as well as life as a breast cancer survivor. In addition, it shows how the Word of God helped me to live through this life-threatening experience. Each chapter also includes words from the Bible that helped me to review my spiritual life, think again what it means to be a follower of Christ, and celebrate God's love for me. Also the dynamics of family, love, the call to communicate and depend on the Word of God, in a simple way have aided in my progress. Prayer, meditation, and studying the Word of God helped to remove my fears, distrust, and filled me with a peace of mind which is unbelievable. I just feel blessed.

Doing something different this time, I did not want breast cancer to treat me, but allow me to treat it. As mysterious as breast cancer is, I did not want it to be to in control. As things occurred, I found ways to deal with them and /or finagle ways to deal when it matters to regain stability. At times, it was draining and burdensome. We were not prepared. My family, friends and I discovered that reflecting and examining how breast cancer impacted me has aided us in our search for stability and wellness.

Dr. Jeremiah Wright, Jr., in one of his sermons said, "Sometimes, God heals our body, and sometimes, he doesn't." This experience can be devastating, but should not be. He reminded us that God is always with us, and that we should learn the difference between what was then and what is now. He reminded us also to get out of the "eight-track mentality" of back then and praise God for what he has done for us. "Receive it and use it." Nearly four years ago, I was diagnosed with breast cancer. During this time, I discovered the dimension of prayers would become my "weapons of mass destruction." Moving ahead, I have learned that prayers, even silent ones, are beautiful and engaging activities that bring peace.

Making a spiritual connection, doing meditation, and studying the Word of God have helped me realize that all things are possible. Sometimes, just the silence helped me to concentrate on God and eagerly anticipate the start of each new phase of my life. Dealing with a new health challenges, at first, my attitude was like a "pebble" in my eye: It hurt at each roll of my eye. Choosing not to look at it this way, but rather as a "stepping stone to higher grounds," removed the "pebbles" of fear, anxiety, and frustration, so that healing could take place. It was amazing how much more positive feelings energized me and changed my way of thinking about my circumstances.

Before my breakthrough, I kept my secret to myself. I did not share the discovery of a lump in my breast with family or friends. You might ask why I did this. Well, for me, at the time, this was just my negative way of thinking. (Or I could say the devil made me do it!) But I have learned this was wrong.

The great Sufi master, Hazrat Inajat Klan's words, "Walking on the turning wheel of earth, living under the ever-rotating sun, man expects a peaceful life" brought a clearer picture to mind. Yes, I was in a season of my life that I thought should be the most "peaceful" time of my life. After thirty-nine years of working, I had finally retired. Family matters were at an all-time high; no one was physically ill or having personal troubles. My son was getting married. I was ready to slow down and travel. Boy, was I wrong! See, these were my plans. Where was God in the scheme of things? Oh, I had my spiritual routines, prayers, and praise, but my agenda was on top. I took it for granted that I could do as I please during this season of my life. I was ready to travel and play.

The discovery of a lump in my breast and all that transpired up to December nineteenth was anything but peaceful. Wrestling with my secret, it was time to reach a place in my life and increase my spiritual development as I sought answers. Saint Jerome said, "Ignorance of the Scriptures is ignorance of Christ." Having a health scare helped me to build up my faith, which broke the devil's hold on me. The life of Saint Anthony is an example of the power of God. In his little brief, it is written:

If you seek for miracles
Death, error, all calamities
The demons fly and leprosy and health succeeds infirmities,

I felt that I was in a tight spot and did not know what to do. Crying out, I asked God to show me what to do. Like Peter, I thought, "Lord, I don't know where to go but you have the words of eternal life." (See John 6:68.) Jesus, the great physician, the mighty healer, and the wonder worker, and invocation of his precious blood are powerful aids to health problems. I was taught by several members of my prayer circles to plead his Blood to flow through every vein to the root of illness. Asking God to reveal what I needed to do as well as his mercy, love and accepting the challenges allowed me to turn to God. It deepened my very steps of spiritual enlightenment. As I prayed for God's strength and solutions for my fears, I did learn not only to listen to the Word of God, but to do what it said without question.

Fighting for my very life made me realize that I was not limited. I had God-given potential. That painful experience became a divine catalyst for spiritual enlightenment and a reminder that God is everywhere. He stands in front of me. He fights for me. He wakes me up in the morning. At night, he puts me to sleep. He has validated me. He grants favor fulfillment and is given authority over my life. I had to learn how to receive what I prayed for, to fast for spiritual encounters, and to do what my parents—who were not able to be here—would have done for me. That is, to pray as only parents can for their child. That is, to pray to receive God's blessings and favors. I was reminded that he is the one who makes a way out of no way, who puts the ones needed at my side, and who can correct any problems I encountered. All this has helped to make my relationship with God much stronger. My real challenge was "to let go and let God," and to move on his own time and not mine.

As I learned about my own ability to commune and be filled with the Holy Spirit, I felt a place of comfort and peace. I know that as long as I seek and follow the Word of God, no matter what is going on in my life, I shall be guided and assisted. That I will feel the love of God as I anticipated a good ending. With the dawn of each new day, I envisioned that I became conscious of my oneness with the universal Spirit of God. As I prayed for guidance, healing, and God's help, I restructured my thoughts to line up with my concept of God and my prayers of the moment. H. Emilie Cady's book, *Lessons in Truth,* teaches that "Every man must take time daily for quiet meditation ... No one can grow in either spiritual knowledge or power without it." On occasions, finding time might seem to be a problem, but everything has a place and a time, therefore, giving God the time that he deserves seemed to be the strategy that worked for me.

No, I did not spend all of my time praying, mediating, or reading the Word of God, but I had always read a lot and on a daily basis. During my radiation treatment, I did have a scare. Noticing that my vision seemed to be blurry, and focusing was hard, I informed my doctor. He explained that the affects of chemotherapy and/or radiation treatment might be causing the problem. He suggested that I not panic and refrain from straining my eyes. Well, I informed him that maybe my eyeglasses needed changing, and that I would make an appointment to get an eye examination. At this point, he suggested that I wait until I had completed my treatment. I agreed to wait until the treatment was over. Spending time with God, I tried the relaxation exercise to keep myself from having negative thoughts. I added St. Lucy to my prayer group, and asked for her intercession on restoring my vision to normal. I still wanted to read, look around, and enjoy this beautiful world, if this was a part of God's plan for me.

This is the prayer in honor of St. Lucy:

> Relying on thy goodness, O God, we humbly ask thee,
> by thy intercession of thy servant, St. Lucy, that thou
> give perfect vision to our eyes that they serve for Thy
> greater honor and glory, and for the salvation of our
> souls in this world, that we may come to the enjoyment
> of the unfailing light of the Lamb of God in paradise.
> St. Lucy, virgin and martyr, hear our prayers and obtain
> our petitions. Amen.
> **(Dominican Sisters of Hope,** *Prayer,* **OUr** *Pathway to God)*

For me, this was an awkward period. Finally, I went to the library and checked out some of the audio materials. This was not the same as reading! At the library, the resource person on the circulation desk was very helpful in putting together a group of material that she thought would help me to enjoy the audio method. Fortunately, I was near the end of my treatment. Calling my optometrist, I scheduled an appointment. By informing the eye doctor of my recent health issues and treatments, he addressed my concerns. My results were music to my ears. My eyes had not been damaged. My vision had changed just a little. Yes, I did need to change my reading prescription. Most of that was due to the length of time since my last prescription, and the aging process. Thanking him for making my day, and moved quickly to select my new frames and process my order. As soon as I returned home, I called the doctor's office and informed him of my happy news. I thanked God for his help. I said to myself, *"All things are possible with God."* For me, it is not just a saying, it is a fact: With God, all things are possible. He is the one who will never leave me. He is the answer to all my problems.

Taking the necessary steps to begin with a clean slate of whatever I needed to get said on this new phase of my life, I decided to focus on reconnecting. Whether it was by making a simple telephone call or by returning books to the library, I needed to get the ball rolling. I embraced the concept that I can have life with breast cancer. I did not dwell on the idea that I cannot live with breast cancer. It was time for me to head into something new. God has brought me to a place where now I want to share my experiences, help others, and testify how wonderful he has been. Sometimes, I used to wonder if it was worth me taking the treatments, keeping the doctors' appointments, and enduring all the changes that I was experiencing, physically and mentally.

Looking back over that phase over my life, I give thanks to God, Mary, my children, my cousin Betty, my family and my friends for not allowing me to give up. If I had to put into words the simplest explanation for all of the growth and success that I have experienced, it would have to be just two word: prayer and obedience. Learning to pray, listening to God, and then doing what he told me to do has not always been easy for me. But learning to apply God's words was like "planting new seeds" which helped me to overcome my fears, anxieties, and frustrations. Personal or public storms, once I have had a "talk with Jesus," I did not feel the same way. This I know! Prayer wheels turning just make things happen and feel right.

I have learned that this mean old disease, with all of its complications, has helped me to develop into a much better—as well as a happier—person. Rushing is no longer on my agenda. Taking the proverbial "time to smell the roses" is high on my list of things to do. This is my vote of confidence for myself. I am going to accept and live the rest of my life incorporating all of my circumstances and outcomes. Because I realized that there will some difficult days, I also believe that, with God's grace, they will all work out fine. The truth is that I do not have to have everything figured out. All I have to do is keep on living and believing in God's words. Proverbs 3:5-6 says, "Lean on, trust in, and be confident in the Lord with all your heart and mind, and do not rely on your own insight or understanding. In all ways, recognize him and he will direct and make straight and plain your paths." With this faith, I have decided that I shall have a whole and fulfilled life, despite the changes of my circumstances and life.

My life has profoundly changed. Every year, on the nineteenth of December, I remember the day when I got a new lease on life. By the Grace of God and a breast cancer experience, a change did take place. This was a painful change. Yes, I did question why I got breast cancer. I tried to live right and eat the right food most of the time. Wondering why this was happening to me, I asked God, "Why? Why would you bring this into my life?" Of course, crying, getting angry, cursing, and focusing on dying are common responses. For me, it became more than that. It was a platform for a better lifestyle of hope, survival, and courage. Spiritually, I have learned that God's words can reveal the secrets to "stepping out of problems into his glory." No matter what I have been through in the past, or what I am going through now, God will deliver me.

Making God my refuge, crying out to him, and declaring his promises, I knew that this adventure could not keep me down. Having breast cancer has made me more alert and aware of how precious my life is. It helped me to believe that "no weapon formed against me shall prosper" (Read Isaiah 14:5-7) and not to forget God's promise in Acts 16:31: "Believe that you might be saved." Why is there a challenge attached to change? Sometimes it was hard to see beyond my circumstances during that awful time, but God showed me a way out. He still had plans for my life. He restored me and strengthened me too. He wanted me to know that "he was not through with me," as Albertiana Walker sings in one of her hymns of inspiration.

Rev. Dr. Wright explained it like this: "God changed your life and your circumstances. For every barrier that has been put up, God sends somebody to help you on your way because he is using you as his instrument." There are methods that are designed to help and protect cancer survivors. There is an old adage, "Cancer changes you." "After facing the disease, many people reshuffle their priorities and alter directions. True, at first, I thought that people will say anything to get attention. After weeks and weeks of thinking about this, I realized that I too could make that statement. It is amazing how powerfully and successfully my brain had returned, despite the chemotherapy and radiation treatments. After riding on the emotional roller coaster of emotions associated with breast cancer, I found it very reassuring to know that my health was stable. There is always a lot to be grateful for. For when I think about how far I have come, medical care, family support, friends, family, and faith are all on my team. Eating better, exercising, a positive attitude and hard work have lifted me up.

Two studies, one in *The New England Journal of Medicine* and the other in the *Journal of the National Cancer Institute,* found a link between physical exercise and a reduction in breast cancer risk. A number of cancer-specific exercise programs, books, and videos are available for those who want to exercise at home or begin a program in their community. Here are just a few:

- *Healing Yoga for People Living With Cancer*
  By Lisa Holthy
- *Focus on Healing Through Movement and Dance: The Lebed Method (www.Focusonhealing.net)*
- *Exercises for Chemotherapy Patients*
  By Harry Raftopoulos, MD and Erin O' Driscoll, RN

"This field is very young and we are seeing benefits and it's time for us to look at other outcome," says Dr. Karen Mustian, Ph.D., an exercise   psychologist and assistant professor of radiation oncology at the University of Rochester Medical School's James P. Wilmot Cancer Center. Before beginning any type of exercises, she recommends that patients check with their doctors. I am still working on my exercise regimen.

To have an ideal life is to have ideal health. Breast cancer has a tendency to snatch this from its survivor, as well as the survivor's family and friends. Spiritually, emotionally, and mentally, a life of wellness aids in the ability to handle life challenges and to transition into triumphs. Striving to discover and take preventive measures as a cancer survivor, so that it does not overtake me and defeat me, has had a lasting effect. Transformation takes time. It does not happen overnight. A song by Heziskiah Walker, "I'm gonna make it. God's gonna bring me through. The devils don't like it. He's mad but I'm so glad that I'm going make it anyhow" really was very uplifting. By transforming my thoughts from negative ones to positive ones, I began a new to restore my health of mind and body. In a copy of *Daily Word,* I read that the first step to healing is letting go of old hurts and mentalities.

Closing my eyes and spending time with God made things easier for me. Thankful for the emotional baggage that I was able to toss out, I was able to spend more time releasing negative thoughts or feelings that were limiting my progress. By reading books, the words of God, articles about breast cancer, or watching television ministries or listening to inspirational music, I went on some incredible journeys. At first, creating friction caused me more frustration, worries, and pain. Once I let go of my private hell and preconceived consequences of the surgery, reconstruction, radiation, chemotherapy, and sought the wisdom and guidance of God, I was prepared for reality again. My despair really had to do with fear. I surrendered and asked God for faith and his unconditional love. The fact that I wanted to live and to be a healthy cancer survivor made my today better than yesterday. Tomorrow will be a better day than today. Rev. Tom Thorpe, an instructor at Unity Institute, teaches that we should "recognize, release and replace. By practicing these steps, we strengthen our awareness of our power of choice and gain greater control over our life experiences."

An affirmation card from *Daily Word* affirms that "through the gentle guidance of the Spirit, I confidently follow new paths."

Reading and compiling the list of scriptures that I have used in this book, I was encouraged to add a prayer after each one of them. Sometimes, as I struggled with doubts and questions, my faith was being tested, but doing reflective readings on the word of God as quoted from my complete Bible kept my mind focused on handling faith and survival as gifts from God. "Making the best of life now and faith in the life to come, I found light guidance and protection by turning to my heavenly father" said John C. Kersten, SVD, in his *Bible Day by Day.* Below is a brief sample of some the scriptures that I have selected to use:

The Lord is my Shepherd; I shall not want...

Psalms 23:1

Loose...and let me go

John 11:43-44

Therefore, do not worry about tomorrow, for tomorrow will take care of itself

Matthew 6:34

Agree with God, and be at peace; in this way, good will come to you.

Job 22:21

What has will be again, what has been done will be done again; there is nothing new under the sun.

Ecclesiastes 1:9

...the peace of God...

Philippians 4:7

If two of you agree on earth concerning anything they ask, it will be done for them by my father in heaven.

Matthew 18:19

Teach me your way, O Lord, that I may walk in your truth, give me undivided heart to revere your name.

Psalms 86:11

... in all your ways, acknowledge him and he will make straight your paths.

Proverbs 3:6

I trust in the power and glory of the Lord with all my heart

Proverbs 3:5

And you will have confidence, because there is hope, you will be protected and take your rest in safety.

Job 11:18

We are writing these things so that our joy may be complete.

John 1:4

Let your steadfast love and your faithfulness keep me safe forever.

Psalms 40:11

For God has not given us the spirit of fear but of power, of love, and a sound mind.

Timothy 1:7

Come to me, all you who labor and are burdened, and I will give you rest.

Matthew 11:28

And we know that all things work together for good of them who love God, to them who are called to his purpose.

Romans 8:28

Rekindle the gift of God that is within you.

II Timothy1:6

The Lord answer you in time of trouble...Give victory to the King.

Psalm 20

Greater is he who is in you than he who is in the World.

John 4:4

All things shall be added unto you.

Matthew 6:33

Surely I am with you always to the end of ages.

Matthew 28:20

While we look not at the things which are seen.

2 Corinthians 5: 18

Somewhere I read that survivors needed to stop talking and planning. It was time to start doing. I needed to stop dreaming about what I wanted to do—I just need to do it! One of the things that I really wanted to do was to move to another location, but in the same village; away from the neighbors from hell. They were literally making my life and existence miserable. I said, "Lord, I come this far and I will not allow them to continue to disrupt my peace of mind." The Spirit spoke to me and asked, "Who told you that you have to take this? Haven't I always been with you? I thanked God, and quickly called my real estate agent and informed him of my decision to place this house on the market and to start looking for me a new home as soon as possible.

After he obtained all of the information that he needed, the house was placed on the market, and a search was on to locate a new one for me. This was another project, but I was up for the task. My family, as well as my friends, knew how unhappy I had become; therefore, they wished me well. For nearly seven months, I would visit available properties in the village. In the fifth month, there was a serious buyer for my place. Praying and talking to God, I said, "You have paved the way for me, now help me to locate a place that you think I deserve." I confidently turned to the Spirit for guidance and fulfillment, and three houses were selected for me to see. My closing on the sold house was near. I prayed that I would locate my new place and relocate before having to pay rent to the new owners. Fighting the foul weather and cold, the real estate agent and I set out to view the latest round of identified homes. I informed the real estate agent that one of these had to be my new home. We stopped to view the first one on the list. No, this was not it. As we drove by the second one, I said there was no sense in wasting our time. As the saying goes, the third one was the charm. Seeing great possibilities in this one, I suggested that we make an offer to the owners. Informing my children, Mary, and Betty of my findings, they all wished me good luck as they added this to our growing prayer list.

Once all the paperwork was completed, the proposal was submitted. Five days later, an affirmative response was rendered. Now the hard work would begin. After I informed Mary, Betty, and my family that we had reached agreement, packing was next on my agenda. Each of them agreed that we needed to plan this event. Betty informed that she would travel to Chicago to help me pack and move into the new house. Oh! At her decision, I was elated. Telephoning Mary and the children to tell them of my additional help, I was literally thinking, "God has opened another door for me." Not only was I surviving—I was *thriving*.

Because I prayed and thanked God for his blessings, once again he had changed my situation. Once the closing date was set, I informed Betty, and she was on her way back. My friends—Mary, the Cades, the Burrises, Clyde, Harold, and Regis—all came and assisted in the move. Of course, the day would not develop without drama. On the day of the big move, the movers did not appear. I thought that I would have the "big one." To make a long story short, I was able to locate movers who could move me that very day. Officially, I was to turn over the keys by seven o'clock. With the help of everyone, we met the deadline. Satan had tried to foil my blessing, but he would not succeed, not this time, because of the many prayer warriors who were on the job. Once we settled, Betty departed for her home. No longer was I in an uncomfortable place. Now I was overjoyed. I thanked God for safely seeing me through this move, challenging experience, and for providing me with such loving friends and family.

No matter what had happened before, this was my time to do some of the things that I wanted to do. There was no putting it off any longer. At my next doctor's appointment, I asked him if it was safe for me to travel. He gave me the okay. With that news, I made plans to visit Betty in Houston, Texas, and then to visit friends and family in my hometown of Opelousas, Louisiana. I was lifted and I felt the wholeness, happiness, and peace. I was not postponing doing anything anymore. Physically and mentally, I had found strength, harmony, and happiness in my life. When in trouble, I no longer have to cry or scream; rather, I acknowledge my relationship with God and repeat that God is.

"Faith…comes through hearing."

(See Romans 10:17.)

Food for Thought

Having breast cancer and the experiences attached to this development have added to my life as a senior citizen. This has not been easy, because this is not what I expected to have to deal with during my golden years. Nevertheless, I am blessed to still be here to testify. What is abundantly clear is that whatever my life presents me with, or wherever my life takes me, I have entered the new world of the cancer survivor, driven by grace and gratitude.

My gratitude is very easy to name:

It is for the life that I now have and for the medical resources that gave me my life back.

It is for my family and friends who have nourished and stood by my side.

It is for the love that I received from family, friends, and my medical team. It is for the opportunity that I have been given to make a difference.

My grace is more intangible, but just as real. It is what I feel from friends, family, and a wider community: their generous support through this experience. It is reflected in my spiritual practices. I needed to tell my story and to care for myself. Once I recognized the limitations of my own body and grant myself the space and time needed to heal all the lessons that I have learned throughout this journey, I could thank God for the incredible team he has placed in my life. The quality of my life is much improved.

Breast cancer is no longer a death sentence. Rather, it is a disease, and if it is treated quickly, the results are encouraging. Mortality from breast cancer has been steadily declining. It is up to each individual woman to continue to seek correct screening and medical attention. Cancer remains a significant health problem for African-American, Hispanic, and American Indian people, despite advances in screening, prevention, and treatment. Women from these populations continue to show an increase with later stages of breast cancer. Research tells us that many American Indians and Alaskan Native tribal languages do not have a word for cancer. In some languages, "cancer" means "something for which there is no cure." Cancer education and dissemination of information to all races and ethnicities is very important. It's all related to the cure of cancer, in addition to the research.

Efforts to estimate the presence of cancer in these populations, until fairly recently, have been complicated by the fact that information and statistics about these groups have not been collected in any comprehensive way until the formation of the Surveillance, Epidemiology, and End Results (SEER) program database, which was expanded to include multiple ethnic groups in the 1990s, as I learned from the Office of Minority Health Resources and Service Administration.

Reading stories of other breast cancer survivors have made me want to know more about how they climbed their "mountains of possibilities." It is my prayer and hope that I would emulate such fortitude going through my own recovery. Wanting to comprehend how they withstood the test of survival, I read every positive article or book on breast cancer that was recommended to me or that I saw in the library or Internet. This was the information that I used in my quest to conquer my fears, depression, and unanticipated circumstances as I sought treatment for breast cancer.

These stories, covering everything from screening to reconstruction to advocacy and the personal experiences of those inspiring women whose lives have felt the impact of the disease, have offered me an insight into this journey that has ultimately brought me such personal peace. Collectively, this is what inspired me to work on this project. This whole experience made me really reflect a lot about life and about how up to that point, I really thought about myself, my life, family, and retirement. This is such a huge way of getting a reality check. Once I began to pray, meditate, and focus positive energy, I got through by realizing the source of strength I needed already existed.

After suffering the physical side effects of chemotherapy and radiation, the support, prayers, and love of family and friends helped me to triumph through these processes. My best medicine was that I did not have to do this alone. Even though I am still on medication, there are some challenges, but with deep faith, family, friends, and my healthcare practitioners, I am still learning to cope and to live my life to the fullest without worrying about every little thing as I get my life back together. As I meet people and struggle to answer their questions about the status of my condition, it feels good that after more than four years of waiting and watching, my life is moving forward again. I still take Arimidex every day to block the production of estrogen.

This experience has been life-altering. When hearing about my experience for the first time, some people say to me, "Oh, I'm so sorry." To them, I respond, "No, don't be sorry. Think of all the good things that God has allowed me to learn in my golden years." Telling myself the truth was a physical thing, developing a better relationship with God was most beneficial. Looking back at my decision to keep my secret was rather foolish, but at the time, it worked for me. The truth is , my moments of indecision stemmed from a fear of the unknown. My fear of not knowing kept me from relying on God and not remembearing what the Lord God had done.(See Psalm 107). Frustrated in this time of difficulty, I prayed that God would bless and bring me to a new place of peace.

In all of my tight spots surgery, reconstruction, chemotherapy and radiation, praying, mediating and relying on the Word of God remained a powerful weapon. By his stripes I have been healed. Invocation of his precious blood is a powerful aid to health. Pleading his precious blood to flow through every vein to the root of my illness, I refused to panic. Jesus is my "health and my healer". Even in the midst of my most difficult situations, I prayed without fail. He provided a breakthrough during my times of uncertainty. Into my life he brought my cousin, Betty, a complete stranger, at one of my weakest times to care for me. One of my dearest friend, Mary, was allowed to start this journey and assisting all my trails without complaining. Lo and behold , he did.

Reading scriptures, praying and meditating have helped me to appreciate who God really is as well as receive the keys to improve my relationship with him. I am still praising him for all that he has done for me and has allowed me to witness. Telling God that I shall continue fighting and praying to live a more righteous life. Wanting to meet his requirements, I have a new determination to " seek first the kingdom of God . . . all things shall be unto you." (See Matthew 6:33)

It is better to trust in the Lord than to put confidence in man.(See Psalm 118:8)

This is the beginning of my story. I have a new sense life, attitude and knowledge of what is important.

So much is happening in breast cancer research now. It is an exciting time. My goal now is to get involved in raising more awareness of the advances in treatment of breast cancer. I became involved with the Jennifer S. Fallick Cancer Support Center because I wanted to join others in supporting breast cancer education. Remembering that God is on my team and makes all things happen, prayer is my first line of defense. Knowing that God loves me, and using that knowledge has made the meaning of my life so much more meaningful. A Yoruba proverb, "No one can uproot the tree which God has planted" has helped this breast cancer survivor to embrace my life, despite my life changes.

Today, allow me to ask you to do two things. Thanks!

First, I want you to challenge yourself to begin living, really *living*. Look for opportunities to bless and serve others. As you press on, stop to look for ways to share and be good to others. By doing this, you will reap the rewards of God's blessings.

Secondly, I want you to go deep within your heart and spirit. You must believe that God's best is available for you. You must believe that he has great things stored for you.

I am unspeakably grateful for all that I have learned and for what I still have yet to learn. I apologize to everyone for the slowness. Yet, I am encouraged by God to grant myself forgiveness for my slowness and not to live in guilt, but to keep trying to get my message out. Thanks for taking the journey with me. Now I pray that you understand why It's *Time to Sing my Song*.

Afterword

Blessed is the man who trusts in the Lord... He is like a tree planted by the water that sends out its roots by the stream.

- Jeremiah 17:7-8

As one person, the number of life-changing events I can experience is limited. Ah, but with the Spirit I can be pulled into deeper explorations and redirect the "creative process." It is simple. I just have to believe, and trust myself. The Science of Mind teaches that "Jesus said that if is done unto you as you believe." No ifs and buts. If is all in what I believe.

Changing my thinking from fear to anticipation of success, things began to change. Remember that you can "change your thinking and change your life". What I thought was my solitary struggle, breast cancer diagnosis, was not. I found scores of people who were willing to work and pray along side me. During my struggles, these families, friends and the words of God changed my thinking and my world. Looking back, I can say that I marvel at my progress, reflect and meditate on the wondrous ways my blessings have made this journey an adventure.

St. Francis of Assisi said, "start by doing what's necessary; then do what's possible. . ." During challenges, it is possible to tap the resources of God which are always available when needed. Being upset by breast cancer, its treatments, pains, or other life related problems, it was comforting to know that right in the midst of my disturbances God was present. Yes, it did take adversity to wake me up to what I took for granted. Today, with faith in God deepen; I refuse to take even the smallest gift of life for granted.

Even though crises and discouragements are part of the human experience, in the course of events, every day is a miracle. On the "eternal frequency of God", the message of God is always being broadcasted; just tune into it. Just put into practice, what you already know; celebrate the oneness with God.

"The Lord is my helper;

I will not be afraid."

- Hebrews 13:5-6

God is with me at all times and in all circumstances. Even when I am faced with what seems like insurmountable odds or events in my life are daunting, God is always with me.

God says:

All things are possible (Luke 18:17)

My grace is sufficient (11 Corinthians 12.9 & Psalm 91: 15)

It will be worth it (Romans 8:28)

I will supply all your needs (Philippians 4-19)

I have not given you a spirit of fear (11 Timothy 1:7)

I give you wisdom (11 Corinthians 1:30)

Cast all your cares on Me (1 Peter 5:7)

I will never leave you or forsake you (Hebrews 13:5)

I will give you rest (Matthew 11: 28-30)

I love you (John 3:16 & John 3:34)

"Life is that ongoing interplay of ups and downs. There is hope for your future, says the Lord."

Jeremiah31:17

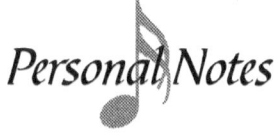

Personal Notes

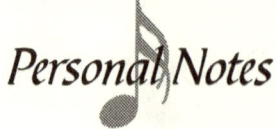

Personal Notes

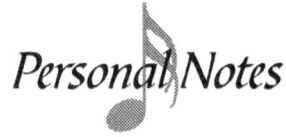

Personal Notes

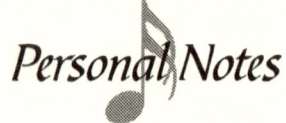

Personal Notes

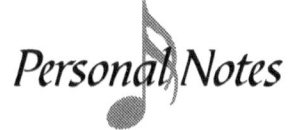

Personal Notes

_____

_____

_____

_____

_____

_____

_____

_____

_____

_____

_____

_____

_____

_____

_____

_____

_____

About the Author

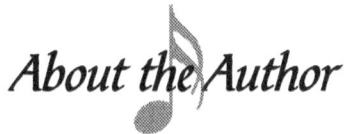

Langston Hughes said it best. "Life ain't been no crystal stair". Between meetings, meals, homework, career, illness and living as a cancer survivor, sometimes it was a struggle to hold on to identity and sanity. With prayer, meditation and looking for divine guidance, M. Marva Allison speaks a message of hope and healing.

M. Marva Allison was born and reared in Opelousas, Louisiana. After graduating from college, Marva took a bold step. To Chicago, Illinois, she relocated to begin her new life as an educator. For thirty-nine years, Marva held many positions as she taught in the Chicago Public School System. Included in her work experience is an Adjunct professor at Prairie State College and Harold Washington College in Illinois. She has taught writing, various literature courses and Adult Continuing Education. Her extensive travels and public appearances have made her an example and inspiration to others. Continuing to volunteer and service others, her spiritual beliefs feed her drives to make life changing decision and win battles. Marva realized that she would not be completely fulfilled until she pursued her dream of embarking on a literary career. Nevertheless, it was not until a few years ago that she placed her fears aside and took her first real step toward venturing into the literary world. Her book is non fiction and inspirational. She is currently working on another motivational book that she hopes to have published soon. Through her volunteering and speaking engagements, she enjoys empowering others.

Marva holds a B.S. in English/French, MA in Administration and Supervision, MA in Cultural Studies: Language Arts and PHD in Education Administration. The mother of one son, grandmother of two, currently lives in a suburb of Chicago, Illinois.

With renewed mind, body and soul, Marva has dedicated time and energy in the quest to make live easier for others.

www.ingramcontent.com/pod-product-compliance
Lightning Source LLC
Chambersburg PA
CBHW031324290526
45784CB00014B/1329